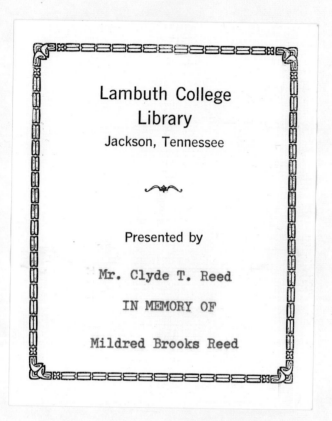

SEEDS OF DESTRUCTION

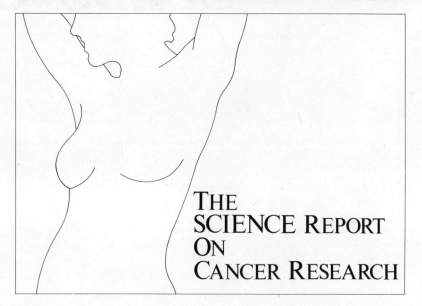

THE
SCIENCE REPORT
ON
CANCER RESEARCH

SEEDS OF

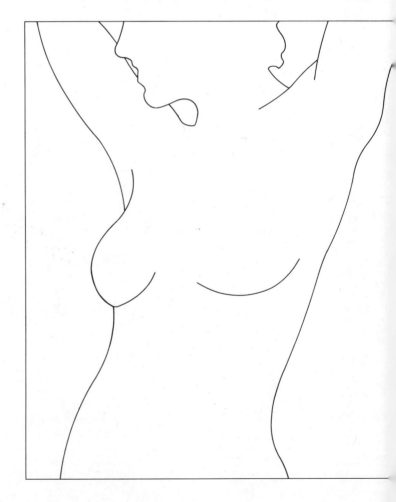

DESTRUCTION

THE SCIENCE REPORT ON CANCER RESEARCH

THOMAS H. MAUGH II
AND
JEAN L. MARX

PLENUM PRESS · NEW YORK AND LONDON

AMERICAN ASSOCIATION FOR THE
ADVANCEMENT OF SCIENCE

Library of Congress Cataloging in Publication Data

Maugh, Thomas H
   Seeds of destruction.

   "Part of the material . . . originally appeared as a series in the
Research News section of Science, the Journal of the American
Association for the Advancement of Science."
   Bibliography: p.
   Includes index.
   1. Cancer. 2. Carcinogenesis. I. Marx, Jean L., joint author. II.
Science. III. Title. [DNLM: 1. Neoplasms—Popular works. 2. Re-
search—Popular works. QZ201 M449s]
RC261.M434   616.9'94   75-15860
ISBN 0-306-30836-3

Part of the material in this book originally appeared as a series in the
Research News section of SCIENCE, the Journal of the American Association
for the Advancement of Science. The authors are members of the
Research News staff of SCIENCE.

© 1975 American Association for the Advancement of Science

Plenum Press, New York is a division of Plenum Publishing Corporation
227 West 17th Street, New York, N.Y. 10011

United Kingdom edition published by Plenum Press, London
A Division of Plenum Publishing Company, Ltd.
Davis House (4th Floor), 8 Scrubs Lane, Harlesden, London, NW10 6SE, England

Preface

There is little prospect of an immediate cure for cancer. The seeds of destruction seem to be sown within all of us, and there is no consensus about how these seeds develop into tumors or about what can be done to halt that development. Indeed, it is often difficult to find a consensus about any aspect of cancer research. The sharply conflicting views of investigators in different subdisciplines has been most aptly summarized by Charles Heidelberger of the McArdle Laboratory for Cancer Research, who argues that "the mechanism of cancer is a mirror into which each man looks and sees himself." This is true despite the fact that large infusions of money and manpower now come to the aid of cancer research.

In late 1974, Betty Ford and Margaretta (Happy) Rockefeller underwent surgery for breast cancer. The extensive publicity surrounding these mastectomies provoked a great deal of interest in the subject of cancer, particularly breast cancer. Newspaper and television stories associated with the operations gave their audiences some insight into the nature of cancer and cancer research, but they provided only a glimpse of the sweeping changes that the directions of cancer research have undergone in the last few years. In large part, these changes simply reflect the natural progression of research, but there is little question that that progression was sharply accelerated by the National Cancer Act of 1971, which initiated what politicians then termed a "crusade against cancer."

As a result of that act, the budget of the National Cancer Institute (NCI) more than tripled, from \$190 million in 1970 to more than \$600 million in 1975. Other sources will probably add half again as much. In

v

1973, the last year for which complete figures are available, NCI's budget of $431 million accounted for some 58 percent of the $752 million available for cancer research and support. Other Federal agencies contributed $90 million, and state and local agencies provided $96 million. Voluntary agencies, primarily the American Cancer Society, contributed $95 million. Private research institutions and industry contributed about $22 million and $17 million, respectively. If the level of support from these other sources remains more or less constant, as is expected, the resources available for cancer programs in 1975 will total more than $920 million—making cancer the best-funded area of biological research in this country.

Meanwhile, in biology there has been increasing emphasis on the study of mammalian cells, rather than on bacteria and other simpler organisms. Hence, with the increased cancer funding and the near-stagnation in support for most other types of biological research, many new investigators have been attracted to the study of cancer. A recent estimate from the National Institutes of Health indicates that some 7.7 percent of the total U.S. biomedical manpower pool—more than 7250 scientists—are working on projects that can be directly related to cancer and many more are working on projects that are peripherally related.

The effect of these stimuli has been to produce distinct changes in emphasis within many of the subdisciplines of cancer research. In viral carcinogenesis research, for example, there has been a subtle shift from efforts to isolate a tangible human cancer virus to more sophisticated attempts to detect biochemical traces of such viruses in human tumors. In chemical carcinogenesis research, there has been a more marked shift away from simple screening and identification of possible carcinogens to a detailed examination of the interaction of chemical and cell. Investigation of the biochemistry of cancer has increasingly been focused on the role of cellular membranes in tumorigenesis and on the identification of tumor antigens that might permit earlier detection and more precise quantification of the disease. And there has been a strong trend in cancer therapy away from reliance on any single tool (such as surgery, irradiation, or drugs) toward a combined-modality approach and a renewed interest in stimulation of the body's own immune defenses.

While no cure is on the horizon and no agreement has been reached on the likely cause or causes of cancer, there has been progress, and there is the promise of much more to come. This book assesses the status of cancer research and examines some of the areas where progress has been most apparent. While it cannot pretend to be either comprehensive or exhaustive, the book focuses on what appears to be some of the most interesting and significant developments in the drive to understand the molecular biology of cancer.

The authors would like to thank Allen L. Hammond and Van R. Potter for their assistance in preparing two of the chapters, Fanny Groom for doing much of the typing, and their colleagues on the staff of *Science* for their enthusiasm and assistance. They would also like to thank Emmanuel Farber, Bernard Roizman, Elizabeth C. Miller, and Herbert Rapp for reviewing parts of the glossary.

THOMAS H. MAUGH II
JEAN L. MARX

May 1, 1975

Contents

List of Illustrations

List of Tables

I
Cancer Etiology

1
What Is Cancer?
How Does It Kill?

Cancer is often thought of as a modern plague caused by pollution, chemicals, and radiation—the byproducts of industrialization—but it may, in fact, be the most ancient of diseases. Its occurrence is recorded in the earliest writings of mankind, but it was not until the 5th century B.C. that Hippocrates first used the Greek word καρκινοσ("crab") to describe the malignancy that spread its pincers throughout the body to choke off life. *Cancer* is the Latin word for crab.

Cancer probably is also the most universal of diseases. It afflicts virtually every species, including plants, but its greatest ravages by far are inflicted on man. On the average, one out of every four individuals will be stricken with cancer; one out of every six will die from it (see Figures 1, 2). In the United States alone, nearly 60 million people now living will be victims of this insidious disease and 40 million of them will die from it. Its importance as a public health problem has grown steadily. In 1900, cancer ranked sixth as a cause of death in the United States; today, it is second only to heart disease.

The Greeks and Romans attributed cancer to a disturbance of the humoral balance of the body, a theory that is not grossly different from some present-day theories suggesting that hormonal imbalances play a major role in its onset. But despite more than 2500 years of observation and research, remarkably little is known about cancer. It is an accepted

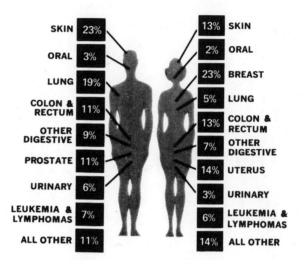

FIGURE 1. Percent of cancer incidence by site and sex.
[Source: American Cancer Society]

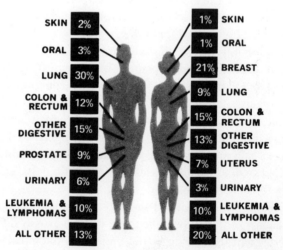

FIGURE 2. Percent of cancer deaths by site and sex.
[Source: American Cancer Society]

fact, for example, that radiation, ultraviolet light, and some chemicals can initiate formation of a tumor, but relatively little is known about the actual mechanism or mechanisms of causation. It is an accepted fact that the biochemistry of tumors is different from that of healthy cells, but relatively little is known about those differences. And it is an accepted fact that as many as half of all cancers can be cured with surgery, irradiation, and chemotherapy, but relatively little is known about the general mechanisms of curing.

It is not even known, in fact, whether cancer is many diseases exhibiting a common pattern of general symptoms or one disease that is manifested in many forms depending, primarily, upon the organ from which it evolves. What is known is that there are more than 100 clinically distinct types of cancer, each having a unique set of specific symptoms and requiring a specific course of therapy. These types can, however, be grouped into four major categories:

Leukemias are diseases in which abnormal numbers of leukocytes (white blood cells) are produced by the bone marrow. This enhanced production resembles the body's normal response to a massive infection, but in leukemias most of the leukocytes do not mature into functional cells. Leukemias are one of the most common malignancies of childhood, but they strike people of all ages. Preliminary results from the National Cancer Institute's Third National Cancer Survey of 1969 suggest that leukemias will account for about 3.4 percent of the 655,000 cases of cancer that will be diagnosed this year.

Lymphomas are diseases in which abnormal numbers of lympho-cytes (a type of leukocyte) are produced by the spleen and lymph nodes. The disease is thus quite similar to leukemia, but in some lymphomas the immature lymphocytes aggregate in the lymphoid tissues. Hodgkin's disease is the best-known form of lymphoma. The cancer survey indicates that lymphomas account for about 5.4 percent of diagnosed malignan-cies.

Sarcomas are solid tumors growing from derivatives of embryonal mesoderm, such as connective tissues, cartilage, bone, muscle, and fat. Leukemias and lymphomas could be considered subgroups of sarcomas, since bone marrow and lymphoid tissues are derived from mesoderm. Sarcomas, leukemias, and lymphomas are the predominant forms of malignancy observed in laboratory animals and in cell cultures, but sarcomas themselves, according to the survey, account for only 1.9 percent of human malignancies.

Carcinomas, solid tumors derived from epithelial tissues, are thus the major form of cancer. Epithelial tissues are the internal and external body surface coverings and their derivatives, and thus include skin, glands, nerves, breasts, and the linings of the respiratory, gastrointestinal, urinary, and genital systems. Carcinomas account for about 85.3 percent of malignancies. (The remaining 4.0 percent of malignancies include tumors derived from mixed tissues, such as ovaries and testes, and all others that are not readily classifiable.)

All of the more than 100 types share three major characteristics that define cancer: hyperplasia, anaplasia, and metastasis. Hyperplasia is the uncontrolled proliferation of cells. Contrary to popular belief, however, hyperplasia does not imply an enhanced rate of proliferation: malignant cells display the same variations of rates as do healthy cells. The malignant cells simply do not respond to the host organism's (as yet unknown) signals to halt division, and thus produce a localized accumulation of tissue.

Anaplasia is a structural abnormality in which the cells resemble more primitive or embryonic cells and in which adult functions are absent or diminished. A malignant lymphocyte, for example, would not retain the capacity to fight infections. Anaplastic cells also lack orientation with respect to the parent tissue: Instead of an orderly spatial arrangement, their distribution is often jumbled.

Metastasis is the ability of a malignant cell to detach itself from a tumor and establish a new tumor at a remote site within the host. This ability reflects both the lessened cohesiveness of cells within a tumor and the capacity of malignant cells to sustain themselves while floating freely in the blood stream or lymph ducts. Unmetastasized tumors can frequently be removed by surgery or irradiation, but there is much less prospect of treating metastasized malignancies.

Cancers are generally not, in themselves, fatal; that is, with rare exceptions, they do not produce toxins, or otherwise kill the host directly. Rather, they seem to have a curious priority on nutrients within the host, nourishing themselves at the expense of other tissues. This malnutrition produces a phenomenon called cachexia, the generalized emaciation and ill-health of the host. Cachexia has frequently been considered to be the ultimate cause of death in a majority of cancer patients, but a recent study suggests that many other factors are involved in such cases.

Julian L. Ambrus and his associates at the Roswell Park Memorial Institute, Buffalo, New York, have studied more than 500 cancer deaths at that institution and found that the chief cause of death was infection, which accounted for 36 percent of the deaths and was a contributory factor in an additional 13 percent. Most of these infections were caused by antibiotic-resistant bacteria. The second most important factors were hemorrhaging and blood clots, which together accounted for 18 percent of deaths and were contributory factors in another 43 percent. Other factors included organ failures caused by invasion by cancer cells, 10 percent; respiratory failure, 19 percent; and cardiovascular insufficiency, 7 percent.

2

Chemical Carcinogenesis

A Long-Neglected Field Blossoms

Chemicals—in the workplace, in the environment, and in the diet—may be the single most important cause of human cancers (Table 1). Many scientists estimate that at least 60 percent and perhaps as many as 90 percent of the 655,000 cases of cancer that will be discovered in the

TABLE 1

Some Chemicals That Are Recognized to Be Carcinogens in Humans
[Source: James A. Miller]

Chemicals	Sites of tumor formation
Certain tars, soots, and oils	Skin, lungs
Cigarette smoke	Lungs
2-Naphthylamine	Urinary bladder
4-Aminobiphenyl	Urinary bladder
Benzidine	Urinary bladder
N,N-bis(2-chloroethyl)-2- naphthylamine	Urinary bladder
Bis(2-chloroethyl)sulfide	Lungs
Nickel compounds	Lungs, nasal sinuses
Chromium compounds	Lungs
Asbestos	Lungs, pleura

United States this year will have been caused by environmental factors, mostly chemicals. Almost 1000 chemicals have been reported to produce tumors in man or other animals, and many times that number are suspect.

Yet despite these statistics, and despite the large amount of effort that has been expended since chimney soot was first identified as a cause of cancer 200 years ago, little is known about the mechanisms of chemical carcinogenesis. In part, this state of affairs results from the greater emphasis that has been placed on viral carcinogenesis. More important, it reflects the fact that, until recently and with only a very few exceptions, the field has been dominated by experimentalists who paint suspect chemicals on the skins of animals or feed the chemicals to animals to determine whether the chemicals induce tumor formation. This process has been useful in identifying carcinogens that should be removed from the environment, but it has been of limited value in elucidating the mechanisms of carcinogenesis or in revealing ways to inhibit or reverse the action of the chemicals.

While a major portion of the resources allotted to the study of chemical carcinogenesis is still devoted to such screening, a new emphasis is being placed on the molecular biology of carcinogenesis. This emphasis has, in the past 5 years, attracted many new investigators to the field and has stimulated a blossoming of research comparable to that in viral carcinogenesis several years earlier. This research already has illuminated some of the first steps in the interaction between carcinogen and cell, has demonstrated that most carcinogens must be activated by the host's metabolism, and has led to the tentative identification of certain groups in the population who may be more susceptible to exposure to carcinogens.

A primary contributor to this blossoming has been the development of cell culture systems in which healthy cells can be transformed (converted to malignant cells) by chemicals. As compared to work in vivo, experiments with these systems provide many advantages: the period between the application of a chemical and the appearance of its effect is sharply reduced; the environment can be totally controlled; host factors can be eliminated; and the dosages of chemicals can be controlled. Most important, the systems permit detailed biochemical examination of the metabolism of the carcinogens and of changes they induce in the cells.

Significantly, it was the development some 5 years earlier of comparable cell cultures which can be transformed by viruses that led to many of the discoveries in viral carcinogenesis.

Maintaining healthy, growing cells in culture, some scientists argue, is in many ways more art than science, a factor that has impeded development and implementation of the culture systems. Regulation of the proper balance of nutrients, serum, and growth factors in the medium is a delicate skill best learned by apprenticeship, and developments in the art are often communicated more readily by personal contact than by journal publication.

The first investigator to apply the art successfully to chemical carcinogenesis was Leo Sachs at the Weizmann Institute in Rehovot, Israel, who developed a hamster embryo cell system in the mid-1960's. This system has been refined and used extensively by Joseph A. DiPaolo and his associates at the National Cancer Institute (NCI) in Bethesda, Maryland. Another early worker in the field was Charles Heidelberger of the McArdle Laboratory for Cancer Research at the University of Wisconsin Medical School, Madison, who developed cell cultures of fibroblasts (connective tissue cells) from mouse prostrate glands. At about the same time, Elizabeth K. Weisburger of NCI and John H. Weisberger of the American Health Foundation in New York City developed cultures of epithelial cells from mouse livers. Several other investigators have subsequently developed systems derived from other types of cells.

The culture systems share the same general characteristics: The parent cells proliferate until they form a confluent monolayer in the culture dish, at which time they stop dividing. Application of appropriate carcinogens produces colonies of morphologically altered cells which do not stop dividing when they contact other cells and which cannot be visually distinguished from malignant cells. The transformed cells acquire antigens and other properties of tumor cells in vivo, but will not grow into a tumorlike mass in culture, partly because of a tumor's requirement for a circulatory system. Because the biochemical characteristics that distinguish malignant from healthy cells are largely unknown, however, the ultimate criterion for transformation is formation of a tumor when the cells are injected into a genetically identical animal or one that has undergone immunosuppression.

Some of the cultures are, by all available criteria, free of oncogenic viruses. Most of the systems are susceptible to transformation by such viruses, but the malignant cells thus formed are antigenically distinguishable from those transformed by chemicals. Some of the cell strains grown in culture are aneuploid; that is, they have an abnormal number of chromosomes, and critics argue that this abnormality creates an intrinsic bias toward transformation. The cultured cells exhibit a very low incidence of spontaneous transformation, however, and the spontaneously transformed cells, unlike those transformed by chemicals or viruses, are generally not antigenically distinct from the parent cells. There is, moreover, a very good correlation between the chemicals that transform cells in culture and those that are oncogenic in vivo.

A crucial reservation in assessing these systems has been that no one has yet satisfactorily demonstrated the transformation by chemicals of human cells in culture. Most of the research findings thus can be applied to humans only by analogy. Another reservation is that many of the cell systems contain only very low concentrations of the enzymes necessary for metabolizing the carcinogens. Perhaps the most important conclusion reached about chemical carcinogens in recent years is that, with a few exceptions, they require activation by the host before they can transform a cell.

A basic principle of chemical carcinogenesis is that a chemical must react irreversibly with cellular macromolecules such as DNA, RNA, or protein to initiate transformation. Several of the known carcinogens, such as β-propiolactone and uracil mustard, are in fact alkylating agents that react readily with nucleosides or amino acids. But the greatest number of carcinogens, perplexingly, are relatively unreactive chemicals, such as polycyclic aromatic hydrocarbons, aromatic amines, and nitrosamines.

Scientists had also been puzzled by the lack of structural or other relationships among the highly diverse carcinogens and by the absence of correlation between carcinogenicity and mutagenicity, another phenomenon that involves interaction of chemicals with cellular macromolecules. These seeming paradoxes have now largely been resolved through the pioneering efforts of James A. Miller and Elizabeth C. Miller of the McArdle Laboratory and the contributions of, among others, Eric Boyland and Peter Sims of the Chester Beatty Research Institute in

London, Bruce N. Ames of the University of California at Berkeley, Charles Heidelberger, Elizabeth and John Weisburger, and Harry V. Gelboin of NCI.

The Millers' widely accepted conclusion is that the form of the chemical that ultimately reacts with cellular macromolecules (the "ultimate carcinogen") must contain a reactive electrophilic center—an electron-deficient atom which can attack the many electron-rich centers in polynucleotides and proteins. Important electrophilic centers include carbonium ions, free radicals, epoxides, some metal cations, and the nitrogen in esters of hydroxylamines and hydroxamic acids. All recognized carcinogens that are not themselves electrophiles are now known or presumed to be metabolized to electrophilic derivatives that are the ultimate carcinogens.

It has thus become clear that the apparent lack of a correlation between the carcinogenicity and mutagenicity of chemicals is because the two activities are measured in different systems. Mutagenicity is generally determined in bacteria, bacteriophages, and yeasts, which usually do not have the enzymes necessary for activation of the carcinogen. In all instances where known ultimate carcinogens have been tested in such systems, however, they have been found to be mutagenic, and it is now becoming generally accepted that all ultimate carcinogens are also mutagens.

The converse of that conclusion appears to be valid too: With the exception of only two classes, all mutagens are generally considered to be carcinogenic. The exceptions are the simple frameshift mutagens, such as acridine ·dyes, that cause mistranscription of DNA by noncovalent intercalation between nucleotides in the double helix, and base analogs, chemicals that can substitute for the purine and pyrimidine bases in DNA synthesis to produce a defective product. Few mutagens from these two classes have been demonstrated to be carcinogenic.

Ironically, the enzymes that activate the carcinogens are those whose primary function is the detoxification and disposal of foreign chemicals. The most important of these are several sets of oxidizing enzymes known collectively as microsomal mixed-function oxygenases. Microsomes are subcellular particles that are, among other things, the seat of protein synthesis. The mixed-function oxygenases are found in moderate concentrations in liver and kidney cells, where foreign chemicals are accumulated, and in variable but generally lower concentrations in most other types of cells.

By oxidizing various functional groups of a foreign molecule, the oxygenases make the chemical more polar—and thus more soluble—and provide a point of attachment for sugars and other molecules that help solubilize the chemical so that it can be excreted. Several other enzyme systems accomplish the same objective in other ways, but the oxygenases have been the most thoroughly studied and are believed to be the most important in carcinogenesis.

One of the best examples of the activity of the oxygenases, unraveled largely by James and Elizabeth Miller, involves the metabolism of 2–acetylaminofluorene (AAF), a potential insecticide that was found during routine biological screening to be a potent carcinogen. Any of the ring carbons of AAF can be hydroxylated by the microsomal oxygenases. The resulting alcohols are esterified with glucuronic acid by a second enzyme to produce a series of relatively inert ring-hydroxy-AAF glucuronides that can be detected in the urines of animals fed AAF. Since identical, synthetically prepared alcohols are substantially less car-cinogenic than is the parent compound, this sequence of reactions is generally accepted to be a detoxification pathway.

One of the oxygenases, however, can also hydroxylate the amide moiety of AAF (Figure 3), and synthetically prepared N-hydroxy-AAF is substantially more carcinogenic than is the parent compound. But N-hydroxy-AAF does not react with cellular macromolecules in culture,

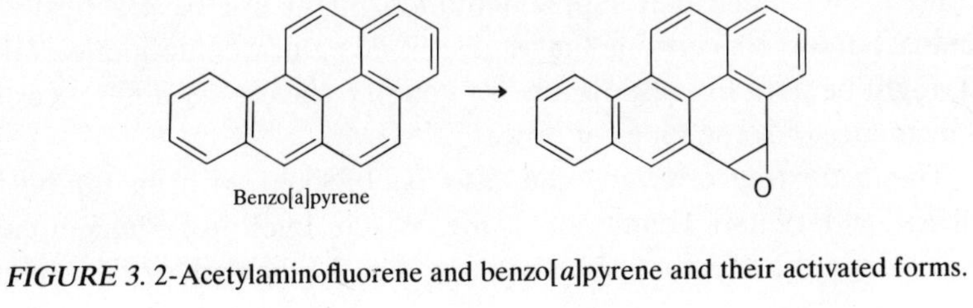

FIGURE 3. 2-Acetylaminofluorene and benzo[*a*]pyrene and their activated forms.

suggesting that it is a metabolic intermediate rather than the ultimate carcinogen. This conclusion was confirmed by the more recent discovery by the Millers and by Charles King of the Michael Reese Hospital and Medical Center, Chicago, Illinois, of a soluble enzyme, sulfotransferase, which converts N-hydroxy-AAF to a strongly electrophilic sulfate ester that is believed to be the major ultimate carcinogen. At least three other pathways for production of electrophilic derivatives of N-hydroxy-AAF have been identified, but they appear to be much less important.

Another good example is found in the metabolism of polycyclic aromatic hydrocarbons such as benzo[a]pyrene, a product of incomplete combustion that is one of the major carcinogens in tobacco smoke. Gelboin has shown that its carcinogenic and toxic effects rely upon its activation by microsomal enzymes. Like AAF, benzo[a]pyrene can be detoxified by hydroxylation of the ring carbons by a subgroup of microsomal oxygenases called aryl hydrocarbon hydroxylases (AHH's). Sims and Gelboin have identified several such metabolites, and suggest that there may be as many as 20, all less carcinogenic than the parent compound. Boyland, Sims and Heidelberger have shown that one AHH in particular can form a reactive epoxide at certain ring positions (Figure 3) to produce what is believed to be the ultimate carcinogen. Some other examples of carcinogens and their metabolically activated derivatives are shown in Figure 4.

Although activation of the carcinogen and its reaction with cellular macromolecules (Figure 5) are only the first of many steps leading to tumor formation, they offer several highly speculative possibilities for moderating the effect of carcinogens. The Millers have found, for example, that flooding the target cell with chemicals that can react with the ultimate carcinogen inhibits the carcinogen's reaction with the cell. Thus, rats fed a diet supplemented with methionine, cystine, or casein have a lower incidence of liver tumors induced by AAF than do those fed a control diet. Such diet supplementation might not be practical for humans, but it is conceivable that undiscerned natural components of the diet might be partially responsible for country-to-country differences in the incidence of some types of cancer.

The activating enzymes can also be blocked with an inhibitor. Gelboin and Leilah Diamond of the Wistar Institute, Philadelphia, Pennsylvania, have found, for instance, that 7,8-benzoflavone inhibits

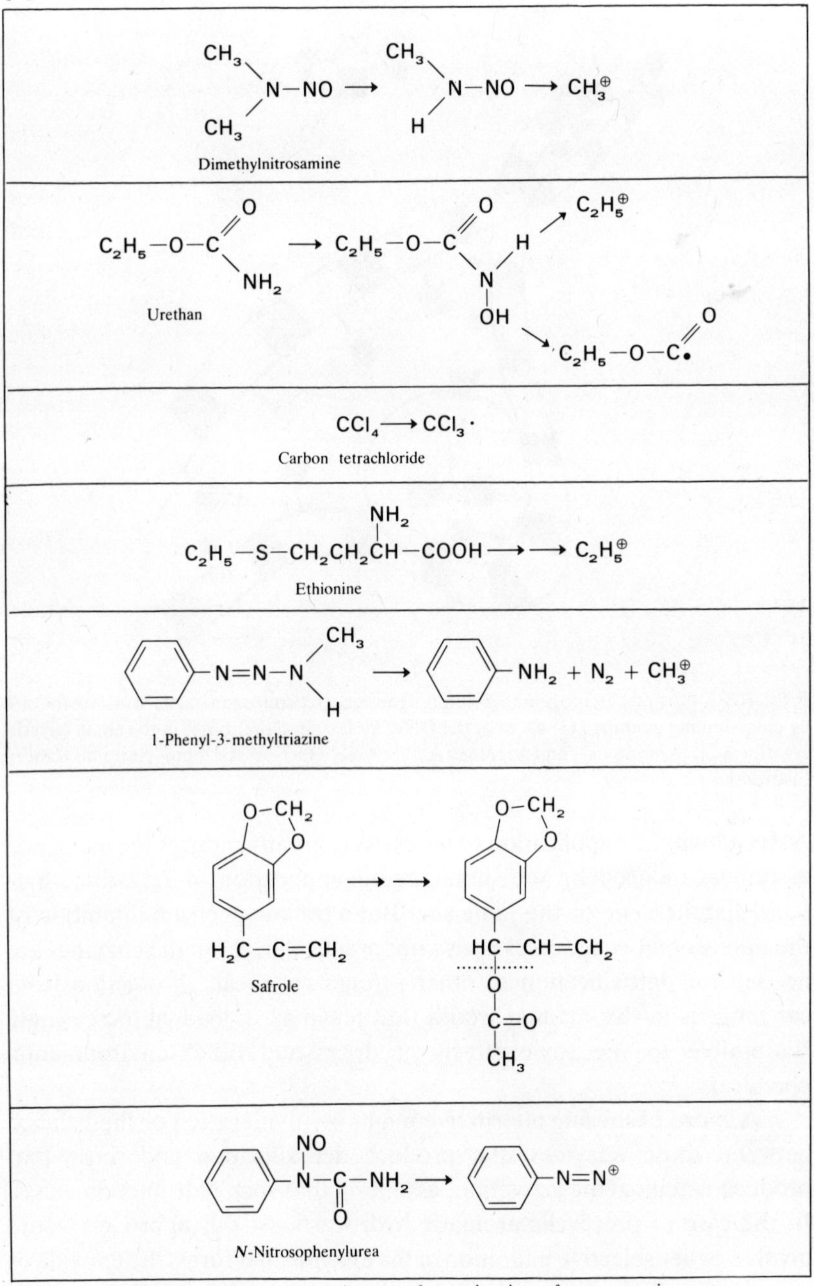

FIGURE 4. The presumed routes for activation of some carcinogens.

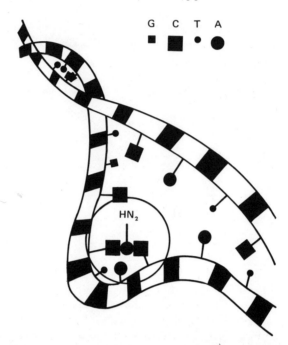

FIGURE 5. Certain carcinogenic alkylating agents, such as nitrogen mustard, act on the cell by cross-linking gaunine (G) bases of the DNA molecule. Other bases in the chain include cytosine (C), thymine (T), and adenine (A). [Source: Harry V. Gelboin, National Cancer Institute]

AHH activity. Its application to mouse skin greatly reduces the incidence of tumors induced by the simultaneous application of 7,12-dimethyl-benz[a]anthracene to the same site. But a broad-spectrum inhibition of the microsomal oxygenases is also not practical because the enzymes are needed for detoxification of other foreign chemicals. Protection from carcinogens in this manner would thus leave an individual increasingly susceptible to the toxic effects of drugs and other environmental chemicals.

A more promising alternative might lie in alteration of the balance between those enzymes that produce detoxification and those that produce carcinogenic activation, assuming that such a distinction exists. In the case of polycyclic aromatic hydrocarbons, this approach would involve either selective inhibition of the enzyme that forms the epoxide or stimulation of the enzymes that hydroxylate the ring carbons. Or if

epoxidation is merely the first step in hydroxylation, as many investigators believe, it might be possible to stimulate the enzymes that convert
epoxides to alcohols. This stimulation is possible because of the well-
documented phenomenon of induction—an increase in the concentration
of the microsomal enzymes in response to exposure of the cell to foreign
chemicals.

A large number of polycyclic aromatic hydrocarbons, drugs, and
other chemicals have been shown to stimulate synthesis of microsomal
oxygenases, but the results of this stimulation can vary greatly. The
Millers, for example, have shown that 3-methylcholanthrene fed to male
rats stimulates ring hydroxylation of AAF, and thus inhibits tumor
initiation by that compound. Stimulation can be a two-edged sword,
however: When the same two compounds are fed to hamsters, *N*-
hydroxylation of AAF is stimulated.

Other enzymes might also profitably be induced. Recent results from
Elizabeth Weisburger suggest that *p*-hydroxyacetanilide reduces the
carcinogenicity of AAF by stimulating the production of enzymes that
convert AAF metabolites to inert glucuronides. But it has by now become
quite clear that the subtlety of the interactions among the various
enzymes makes manipulation of their activities a delicate task that will
require a great deal more knowledge before it is attempted in humans.

The greatest benefit from the oxygenases, in fact, might come from
using them to identify individuals who should limit their exposure to
certain types of carcinogens. The capacity for enzyme induction is not
uniform, so some individuals have a greater capacity than others.

Gelboin and Charles R. Shaw of the M. D. Anderson Hospital and
Tumor Institute, Houston, Texas, have recently demonstrated that AHH
activity can be identified and quantified in lymphocytes from human
blood—the first reports of the presence of this enzyme in an easily
obtainable human tissue. The concentration and inducibility of AHH in
the lymphocytes presumably correlates with those characteristics in other
tissues such as the lung, where AHH is believed to activate the carcinogenic hydrocarbons in tobacco smoke.

Shaw's preliminary results suggest that about 9 percent of the white
population in the United States has the capacity for induction of high
concentrations of AHH; moderate concentrations can be induced in
about half of the others, and only low concentrations in the rest. His initial

findings also indicate that the incidence of lung cancer is about 36 times higher in cigarette smokers with high AHH inducibility than in those with low inducibility, and about 16 times higher in cigarette smokers with moderate AHH inducibility. If this postulated relationship between high AHH inducibility and increased lung tumor incidence can be substantiated, and if the lymphocyte assay can be proved and adapted for large-scale use, then it might for the first time be possible to identify individuals who are at a greater risk from smoking and who should thus be given the greatest encouragement to quit.

Factors other than the microsomal enzymes probably also influence the interaction of carcinogen and cell, but very few have yet been identified. Vitamin A is one of the important factors that has been recognized. Working with hamster tracheas in organ culture, Michael B. Sporn of NCI has shown that the percentage of added benzo[a]pyrene that becomes covalently bound to epithelial cell DNA is much higher in tracheas from vitamin A–deficient animals than in those from healthy specimens. The tracheas cannot be maintained in culture long enough to ascertain whether the increased binding is associated with an increased incidence of tumor formation, but all evidence suggests that the association exists.

Sporn's observation is one of the first reports of a carcinogenic response associated with a nutritional deficiency. More important, vitamin A deficiency is a common one. Barbara A. Underwood of the Columbia University School of Public Health and Administrative Medicine, New York City, has performed analyses which suggest that 15 to 30 percent of the U.S. population suffers from long-term vitamin A deficiency without overt symptoms. Since there is no evidence that the induction of microsomal enzymes is associated with vitamin A concentrations, it thus appears that individuals with vitamin A deficiency form a second population subgroup that is more susceptible to carcinogens in tobacco smoke. Presumably, then, the greatest incidence of lung cancer might be found in cigarette smokers who have high AHH inducibility and who are deficient in vitamin A.

Beyond the stage of the carcinogen's activation and interaction with cellular components, very little is known about the course of chemical carcinogenesis. The main theories can be divided into two broad categories, genetic and epigenetic. Postulated genetic mechanisms include modification of existing DNA; modification of RNA, which is subsequently transcribed into DNA that is integrated into the host DNA; and modification of proteins to decrease, at least temporarily, the fidelity of copying DNA. The most reasonable theory of epigenetic mechanism is based on protein alterations that effect quasi-permanent changes in the transcription of DNA (that is, gene expression). This process is analogous to the (unknown) mechanism by which a change in gene expression converts embryonic cells into mature cells characteristic of a specific organ.

An alternate epigenetic mechanism involves alterations of proteins in individual cells or in the immune system that might allow preferential proliferation (selection) of previously existing malignant cells. Many carcinogens are, in fact, also immunosuppressants. Recent evidence from Gelboin's laboratory, moreover, indicates that some of the carcinogen-activating enzymes are present and highly inducible in tissues involved in immunological activity. Interaction of the ultimate carcinogen with these tissues could produce immunity impairment without being carcinogenic in itself.

Heidelberger, however, has demonstrated that single mouse prostrate cells in culture can be transformed by 3-methylcholanthrene with a high efficiency. This result suggests that selection probably is not a primary mechanism for chemical carcinogenesis, although it may well play a secondary role in promoting tumor growth or in the cocarcinogenesis of chemicals and viruses. Heidelberger has also shown, in collaboration with Robert Nowinski of McArdle Laboratory, that carcinogens do not transform the prostate cells from some strains of mice by activating a latent oncogenic virus, eliminating that possibility as an epigenetic mechanism.

There is little conclusive evidence to support either a genetic or an epigenetic theory. But many investigators, typified by Emmanuel Farber of the Temple University School of Medicine, Philadelphia, Pennsylvania, favor a genetic explanation because a modification of existing DNA is the simplest possible mechanism and because such an explanation provides a straightforward analogy to mutagenesis. Perhaps most important, Farber argues, modifications of DNA provide the most rational explanation for preservation of necessary information during the prolonged period between application of the carcinogen and appearance of a tumor. This latent period is typically between 10 and 20 percent of the host's life-span, and it is difficult to visualize retention of simple protein alterations during such an extended period.

It is in elucidating the mechanisms of tumor development during this latent period that cell culture systems offer the most promise, and it is for that reason that most investigators consider them so important. But in view of the complexities involved, it may be quite some time before those mechanisms are revealed.

Since it is not yet possible to reverse the carcinogenic effects of chemicals in man, a major facet of research in chemical carcinogenesis has been the prevention of exposure by identifying carcinogens and removing them from the environment. Efforts to control recognized carcinogens have met with mixed results—witness the 10 percent increase in U.S. cigarette consumption during the 10 years since the U.S. Surgeon General's report which linked smoking and lung tumors—but their identification has continued at a modest rate.

Nearly 450 chemicals are now being screened for carcinogenicity at 28 different U.S. laboratories under the sponsorship of the NCI carcinogenesis program. This screening is expensive and time-consuming. Each chemical tested requires, on the average, 3 years, 500 animals, and $70,000. Moreover, only a fraction of the available chemicals can be tested. Even if all the screening facilities in the country were mobilized, by one estimate, it would still be possible to screen only about 700 chemicals per year. At that rate, it would take many years to screen all the new chemicals that are introduced in any one year, and a much longer time to screen all those already in the environment.

A promising solution to this problem is to be found in cell culture systems. Use of these systems could sharply reduce the time and expense of screening. Morphological changes indicative of carcinogenicity appear in cultured cells as soon as 2 weeks after application of a chemical, and confirmation that the altered cells cause tumors in animals usually requires no more than 18 weeks. A substantial effort thus being made to refine the systems for use in screening.

Many investigators are examining this approach, but their work is typified by that of Roman Pienta and his associates at NCI's new Frederick Cancer Research Center in Frederick, Maryland. Pienta's group is now about halfway through a 2-year project to develop standardized cell strains and assay techniques that will make it possible to compare results obtained in different laboratories. The cell strains they are examining are the hamster embryo cell cultures developed by Leo Sachs and refined by Joseph A. DiPaolo. Most of Pienta's effort now is being devoted to screening about 100 chemicals whose carcinogenicity is well defined to ensure that the tests do not produce misleading results. His group is also developing stringent criteria for determining whether the test cells have been transformed. If this phase is successful, the cultures and techniques will be made available to other investigators.

Even with success, however, a major problem remains: The hamster cells contain insufficient concentrations of some of the enzymes known to be necessary for activation of most carcinogens. Investigators are thus looking for some way to expose the chemicals to these enzymes before or during the screening.

One approach adopted by Pienta and others relies on liver cells—which have relatively high concentrations of the necessary enzymes—that have been x-irradiated so they can no longer proliferate. The liver cells could thus be added to the cell cultures and presumably would metabolize the test chemicals without interfering with the screening. Insufficient results have been obtained for a proper assessment of this scheme.

An alternative approach, developed by DiPaolo, requires injection of the chemical into a pregnant hamster. The hamster fetuses, which are thus exposed to both the chemical and its metabolites, are subsequently removed, and embryonic cells from them are cultured in the same manner as those in the fibroblast system. DiPaolo has tested 12 carcinogens and 5 noncarcinogens in this fashion with no false negatives or false positives, so the testing is being expanded to include more chemicals.

Perhaps the most promising approach of all has been adopted by Bruce N. Ames and his associates at the University of California at Berkeley. Because all known carcinogens have been shown to be mutagens also, Ames argues that a bacterial test for mutagenicity would provide a rapid, inexpensive test for carcinogenicity. He has developed a set of four mutant strains of *Salmonella typhimurium* that revert to the wild type strain in the presence of all carcinogens with which they have been tested. The bacterial strains do not respond to those carcinogens that must be activated by mammalian metabolism, but Ames says this problem can be overcome by growing the bacteria in the presence of a homogenate of rat or human liver tissue. NCI is currently sponsoring research to confirm the utility of this approach.

These or similar systems might finally make it possible to screen all new chemicals before their introduction, but there is one more reservation. The results obtained in animal cells can be applied to humans only by analogy and, while these analogies have generally been good, they are not perfect. The ultimate test, still out of reach, would thus be based on cultures of human cells.

3
Viral Carcinogenesis
Role of DNA Viruses

Scientists have grappled with the idea that viruses could cause human cancer for at least 70 years, but only within the last 10 years have they accorded it widespread respectability. The idea was suspect for so long because cancer in humans simply did not behave like other diseases of viral origin. It did not appear to be infectious, and there were no confirmable isolations of a causative virus. During that time, however, a comparative handful of pioneers accumulated evidence that proved that viruses did in fact cause cancer in animals. So the recurring question was: If viruses can cause cancer in animals, then why not in humans?

The concept that viruses can cause cancer is attractive for two reasons. First, introduction of viral DNA or RNA—and thus of new genetic information—into cells can account for their permanent transformation to the malignant state. Second, identification of a viral cause for a cancer may permit the development of a vaccine to prevent and ultimately eradicate the disease, just as vaccination has virtually eliminated smallpox in the United States. Given the dread with which people view cancer—an attitude that may have contributed to earlier reluctance to consider that cancer had a viral etiology and might be contagious—the prospect of a vaccine is indeed a heady one.

Because the disease called cancer is actually a number of different diseases, demonstration of viral involvement in the etiology of one type of cancer, or of several types, does not mean that the problems of cancer etiology will be solved. According to some estimates, the majority of cancers may be chemically induced. Alternatively, the virus may be a necessary but not sufficient contributor to development of cancer. Other factors, such as genetic disposition, immunological deficiency, or exposure to chemicals or radiation, may also be needed. A requirement for two or more causes, acting together in the proper sequence, may help to explain why—if viruses are involved—there is little evidence that cancer is contagious.

Interest in the DNA viruses as human cancer virus candidates at first centered on the adenoviruses and papovaviruses. Adenoviruses, which cause respiratory infections in humans, and papovaviruses, such as SV40 and polyoma virus, produce tumors in experimental animals and transform animal cells in culture. But despite the fact that they are widespread, there are few indications that they are implicated in human cancers. Adenoviruses and papovaviruses have served as valuable tools for studying malignant transformation in the laboratory.

During the mid-1960's, however, the herpesviruses, a family of complex DNA viruses (Figures 6 and 7), attracted the attention of a number of investigators who were seeking to establish a link between

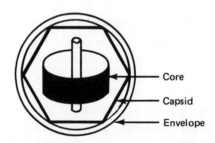

Core

Capsid

Envelope

FIGURE 6. Schematic representation of the structure of herpes simplex viruses. These complex viruses have diameters ranging from 150 to 200 nanometers and molecular weights of about 1 billion. The complete particle contains an inner core consisting of DNA coiled in the form of a doughnut; proteins arranged in the shape of a barbell pass through the hole. The core is surrounded by a capsid composed of layers of proteins. The capsid is in turn enclosed in a membranous envelope containing viral glycoproteins. So far, about 50 proteins, synthesized in infected cells under the direction of viral DNA, have been identified. Of these, at least 27 are structural proteins of the virus. [Source: Adapted from a diagram by Bernard Roizman, University of Chicago, Illinois]

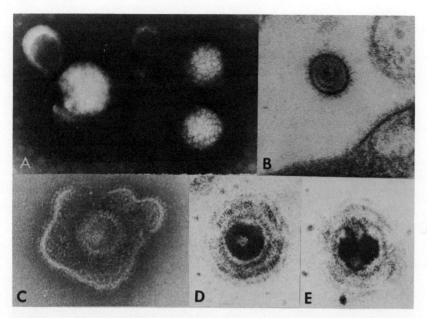

FIGURE 7. Electron micrographs showing different views of the HSV I virion. (A) Negative stain of the intact virion (left) and two capsids (right). The proteins of the outermost layer of the capsid are arranged in an icosahedron containing 162 structural subunits, or capsomeres. (B) Thin section of an extracellular virion showing spikes on the membrane. (C) Negative stain of an HSV I virion with a broken envelope. The stain has penetrated to show the capsid and tegument (an amorphous protein material between the capsid and envelope). (D and E) Thin section of HSV I virions showing doughtnut-shaped core in two different orientations. [Source: Bernard Roizman]

cancer and viruses. The lines of evidence for such a connection now stretch from several laboratories. They point to at least three herpesviruses that may be involved in human cancers and also to several that cause cancer in animals and may serve as models for studying human disease.

Proving that a virus causes human cancer has been so difficult because Koch's postulates—which have served for almost 100 years as the criteria for establishing that a disease is caused by a given infectious agent—cannot be fulfilled. One postulate requires the isolation of the agent from all infected organisms. But viruses cannot be seen in fresh human tumor cells, nor can infectious particles be recovered from them. Although this complicates proof of a causal relationship, it is not surprising because when DNA viruses such as herpesviruses reproduce in cells they kill them—a consequence that is necessarily incompatible with development of cancer. Only after "tricks" have been perpetrated on tumor cells—such as culturing them, sometimes with other kinds of cells—can an infectious virus be demonstrated. This raises the possibility that the virus is a contaminant. Another postulate requires an experiment that cannot be performed on humans with a suspected oncogenic virus: induction of the disease in a suitable animal by a pure preparation of the agent.

Thus investigators must rely on indirect or circumstantial evidence to prove their case against herpesviruses. Their strategies include epidemiological studies, now usually done in conjunction with immunological studies to determine whether the virus has left traces of its presence in the form of antibodies against it in the patient's blood; study of tumor cells to detect the presence of viral DNA or RNA or of virus-associated antigens; comparison with virus-induced animal tumors; and study of the oncogenic potential of the virus in both cultured cells and in living animals, especially nonhuman primates.

Since 1964 when M. A. Epstein and Y. M. Barr discovered a virus in cultured Burkitt's lymphoma cells, this herpesvirus—now called the Epstein-Barr virus (EBV)—has been a prime candidate as a human cancer virus. Burkitt's lymphoma is a cancer of the lymphoid system that afflicts children in certain areas of Africa and New Guinea. Among the investigators who have studied EBV, frequently in collaboration, are George Klein of the Karolinska Institutet, Stockholm; Werner Henle and Gertrude Henle of the University of Pennsylvania Medical School, Philadelphia; George Niederman of the Yale University School of Medicine, New Haven, Connecticut; Paul Gerber and Gary Pearson, both at the National Cancer Institute (NCI), Bethesda, Maryland; and Dharam Ablashi of the NCI Frederick Cancer Research Center, Frederick, Maryland.

Like the other herpesviruses, EBV is widely disseminated in the human population. In studies conducted in areas of Africa where Burkitt's lymphoma is endemic, up to 90 percent of the children had antibodies to EBV before the age of 2 years. But the virus is not restricted to Africa. In the United States, approximately 75 percent of the population acquires antibodies before adolescence. Early infection usually produces no characteristic illness. EBV has been closely associated with Burkitt's lymphoma, a cancer of the lymphoid system, and with nasopharyngeal carcinoma. The same virus, or one so closely related to it that they cannot be distinguished by current techniques, causes infectious mononucleosis, a disease whose symptoms may mimic those of leukemia except that mononucleosis is self-limiting and relatively mild.

Most of the evidence now linking EBV to human cancer relates to Burkitt's lymphoma. Investigators have detected a number of distinct, EBV-related antigen-antibody systems that can be used as indicators of viral involvement in Burkitt's lymphoma and that may reflect the progress of the disease. For example, patients with Burkitt's lymphoma have eight to ten times as much antibody against viral capsid antigen (the capsid is the protein layer surrounding the DNA core of the virus) as do normal controls. Although EBV is common, Burkitt's lymphoma is rare. According to Werner Henle, a prospective study now under way should determine whether the children who develop Burkitt's lymphoma are among those few who escape early infection (a situation analogous to that thought to pertain to infectious mononucleosis) or whether the disease occurs only rarely, for unknown reasons, among those who were infected in infancy.

Antibodies to another EBV-related antigen complex, called early antigens because when cultured cells are infected with EBV they appear early in the virus replication cycle, are rarely seen in healthy people but attain high concentrations in patients with Burkitt's lymphoma. These antibodies could be used to predict the probable course of the disease. Patients in whom the antibodies disappeared or declined after chemotherapy became long-term survivors—living 5 to 10 years without a relapse. If the antibody concentration did not decline, the prognosis for the patients was generally poor. Investigators think it unlikely that antibodies to a passenger virus (one that just happened to be present but was not causative) would be of prognostic value.

Although EBV particles are not found in Burkitt's lymphoma cells removed by biopsy, other traces of the virus can be detected. These include certain EBV-associated antigens and also viral DNA. Cellular DNA hybridizes either with viral DNA or with RNA transcribed from viral DNA. The results of the hybridization experiments indicated that each lymphoma cell contained multiple copies of EBV DNA. No one knows why the viral DNA is not completely expressed in tumor cells. It may be defective or partially repressed. A small number of cells in a few cultured cell lines derived from biopsied tumor cells did produce infectious viral particles or incomplete noninfectious particles. All of the cells, however, produced an EBV-associated nuclear antigen that may be analogous to the T (tumor) antigens produced in cells infected by oncogenic animal viruses such as SV40.

Another indication of the oncogenic potential of EBV is its capacity to transform lymphoid cells in culture. Normal lymphoid cells do not proliferate in culture and die out after a short time. Transformed cells, which harbor the viral genome, do grow in culture, and they have the characteristics usually associated with transformation, including loss of density-dependent inhibition of growth.

Production of cancer in laboratory animals with EBV would provide additional evidence that it causes related disease in humans, and would also provide a model system for studying therapeutic techniques. George Miller and his colleagues at Yale University induced lymphomas in a small number of marmosets by inoculating them with materials containing EBV. Although Miller has not conclusively proved that EBV itself caused the tumors, similarities between the human disease and that in marmosets make this the most likely explanation.

Herpesvirus saimiri, an oncogenic virus of nonhuman primates, may provide another model for investigating human lymphomas. This virus causes no overt disease in its natural host, the squirrel monkey, but induces lymphomas or occasionally lymphocytic leukemia in marmosets and owl monkeys. The behavior of the virus resembles that of EBV, both in its effects in living animals and in cultured cells. For example, neither EBV nor herpesvirus saimiri particles can be demonstrated in biopsied tumor cells but they are occasionally produced in cultured cells. Moreover, the antigen-antibody patterns associated with the latter virus resemble those of EBV.

Evidence implicating the herpes simplex viruses I and II (HSV I and HSV II) in the etiology of human cancer is similar to that outlined for EBV. Investigators have elucidated a series of correlations between certain types of cancer and past infections with the viruses, the presence of antibodies to virus-associated antigens, the presence of virus-associated antigens in tumor cells, and, in one case, the presence of viral

DNA in tumor cells. The herpes simplex viruses also transform cells in culture.

These viruses are again familiar human pathogens. Herpes simplex virus I primarily infects regions around the lips (where it causes the common "cold sores"), the oral cavity, and the eyes. Herpes simplex virus II usually infects genital areas and is transmitted venereally. Both may persist in the host for long periods of time and produce recurrent infections.

Beginning in the mid-1960's, epidemiological studies such as those conducted in the laboratories of André Nahmias at the Emory University School of Medicine, Atlanta, Georgia, Laure Aurelian at Johns Hopkins University School of Medicine, Baltimore, Maryland, and Joseph Melnick at Baylor College of Medicine, Houston, Texas, implied an association between HVS II, which Nahmias had identified as the cause of up to 95 percent of genital herpes infections, and cancer of the uterine cervix. Both conditions were correlated with increased numbers of sexual partners for the women surveyed. Women with cervical cancer had higher frequencies of antibodies to HSV II than did controls.

The problem with interpreting these results is that women likely to contract one veneral disease, genital herpes, might also be likely to acquire the other, cervical cancer. In other words, the two conditions could be independent consequences of a high degree of sexual activity. The solution to the problem requires close matching of women with cervical cancer and control women with regard to age, race, socioeconomic status, and all the variables indicative of sexual activity.

In one such study with carefully matched women, William Rawls, in Melnick's laboratory, found that women with antibodies to HSV II had a risk of acquiring cervical cancer more than twice as great as that of women without antibodies. There was no greater incidence of breast cancer in women with antibodies than in women without. Melnick concluded that the risk of developing cervical cancer appeared to be more closely related to HSV II infection than to attributes associated with the number of sexual partners.

Virtually all epidemiological studies conducted to date have been retrospective ones in which the information about herpes infection was gathered after the onset of cancer. Nahmias and his associates are currently conducting a prospective study, begun in 1963, to determine whether women who have had genital herpes infection or who have antibodies to HSV II develop more cervical cancers than women who do not have the antibodies. The long latent period of cancer and the need to include large numbers of carefully matched women compound the difficulty of such studies. Nahmias' preliminary results indicate that women with antibodies to HSV II do have a higher incidence of cervical cancer than do women without antibodies. Women who were pregnant when genital herpes was diagnosed had an even higher incidence. Nahmias is now investigating whether changes in the female genital tract during pregnancy may predispose to initiation of cancer by HSV II.

Malignant transformation of cells by viruses probably depends on expression of some viral gene or genes. Consequently, investigators have been looking for viral gene products, both as indicators of the virus presence and as possible causes of transformation. Nonvirion antigens (antigens coded by the viral DNA but not themselves part of the viral particles) attracted quite a bit of attention in April, 1973, when Albert Sabin announced that he and Giulio Tarro of the University of Naples, Italy, had found antibodies to these antigens in blood serums from patients with a number of cancers, principally those of the mouth, throat, and urogenital regions, but not in the serums of a large number of control patients.

Since then Sabin has been unable to replicate the experiments and subsequently announced that he was withdrawing the data. Tarro, however, apparently stands by his contribution to the collaboration, for his name did not appear on the retraction. Thus, the status of this work remains unclear.

Other investigators have found evidence of nonvirion antigens in human tumor cells. According to Ariel Hollinshead of the George Washington University Medical School, Washington, D.C., and Tarro, soluble cell membrane antigens extracted from carcinomas of the lip and of the uterine cervix reacted with antibody to HSV nonvirion antigens. Soluble antigens from an intestinal tumor or from normal vaginal tissue did not react with the antibody in the immunological assay. Thus, it appeared that lip and cervical carcinomas contained HSV nonvirion antigens not found in normal tissue or an unrelated tumor.

Researchers hope that they can monitor the effectiveness of cancer treatment by measuring the concentration of antibodies against virus-associated antigens. Hollinshead and her colleagues found that 70 to 90 percent of the patients with carcinomas of the head, neck, or uterine cervix had antibodies to HSV nonvirion antigens. Removal of the tumors might be expected to remove the antigen source with subsequent disappearance of the antibodies against it. But Hollinshead and Tarro, in a collaborative study with Rawls and Paul Chretien of NCI, found that individuals who had no clinical signs of carcinoma after successful treatment still retained antibodies to HSV antigens.

Hollinshead does not know why the antibodies did not disappear. She points out that the results parallel those of Chretien and his colleagues. They found that individuals cured of certain carcinomas still had deficient cellular immune responses, while individuals cured of other types of cancer did not have impaired cellular immunity. Hollinshead hypothesizes that herpes simplex viruses may themselves suppress the activity of the immune system. Alternatively, the immune defect may be a preexisting condition that contributes to cancer development.

Antibodies to other antigens (apparently not the same as the nonvirion antigens studied by Hollinshead) associated with HSV II do appear to correlate with the clinical state of patients with cervical cancer. Aurelian and her colleagues found that cultured human epidermoid carcinoma cells infected with HSV II produce an early antigen (or antigens) that reacts in an immunological assay with antibody in serums from patients with cervical cancer. There was no reaction with serums from normal controls or from patients with other cancers, including carcinomas. The presence of the antibody correlated well with the extent of the disease. Of patients with invasive cancer, 91 percent had antibody to the antigen, but only 35 percent of patients with very early cancerous changes had it.

Moreover, the antibody may be of prognostic value. Aurelian and her colleagues did not detect it in 22 patients who had had invasive cancer but who were free of the disease after treatment. They also studied four patients in whom antibody had been detected prior to treatment; in the 2 years after radiation therapy, antibody was found in the two individuals whose cancer recurred but not in the two who remained free of clinical symptoms.

Finally, Gilbert Chiang, in Nahmias' laboratory, has recently detected herpesvirus nuclear antigens in biopsies of invasive cervical cancers. Thus, there is evidence that at least three groups of HSV-associated antigens—nonvirion, early, and nuclear—are found in cervical cancers.

Virus-associated antigens are not the only traces of herpesviruses detectable in cancer cells. Bernard Roizman and his colleagues at the University of Chicago, Illinois, detected fragments of HSV II DNA in one specimen of human cervical cancer tissue. In contrast to Burkitt's lymphoma cells, which contain multiple copies of the EBV genome, the tumor cells contained about 40 percent of the HSV II genome. According to Roizman, only 5 percent of the HSV genome was transcribed into RNA in the tumor cells while approximately 50 percent is transcribed when the virus reproduces in and kills cells. These findings support the hypothesis that transformation is effected by defective viruses, possibly when they are integrated into the cell genome. Roizman and his colleagues are using hybridization techniques to determine whether different cervical tumors contain common DNA sequences whose expression is required for transformation.

It appears that inactivated or defective herpesviruses can transform cultured cells. Infectious particles reproduce and thus kill the cells by lysing them. Fred Rapp at the Milton S. Hershey Medical Center of Pennsylvania State University, Hershey, found that HSV I and HSV II transformed hamster embryo cells after the viruses had been inactivated photodynamically. Photodynamic inactivation involves treating the virus first with a dye, then with light. When the dye forms a complex with viral DNA, subsequent absorption of light energy causes a reaction that damages the DNA and results in loss of infectivity. Rapp and others have shown that HSV I and II, inactivated by ultraviolet light, also transform hamster cells.

Because of his results, Rapp has expressed concern about the use of photodynamic inactivation for treating recurrent genital herpes infections. Such treatment is frequently successful, but Rapp suggests that it is potentially hazardous if inactivated HSV is indeed carcinogenic. He thinks that use of the treatment should be suspended until its oncogenicity can be determined in animals.

A large percentage of the human population has been exposed to one or more of the herpesviruses, yet relatively few get cancer. Most investigators think that other factors—in addition to DNA viruses—must contribute to initiation of the disease. Of prime interest is the role of the immune system. The immune system is generally thought to prevent tumor development by detecting tumor cells—because of their tumor- or virus-associated antigens—and destroying them. A deficiency in the immune system, whether the result of a genetic defect, infection, or immunosuppression (as in transplant patients who suffer an increased cancer incidence), could therefore contribute to cancer development.

Another puzzling problem is the latency of the herpesviruses. Although the viruses kill infected cells when they reproduce within them, HSV I and II can survive in the host for long periods without causing clinically obvious disease and apparently without provoking an immune attack. Recurrences of active infection do happen when the latent virus receives appropriate stimuli, including psychological upsets. A number of investigators, such as J. G. Stevens of the University of California School of Medicine in Los Angeles, think that the viruses are maintained without reproducing in certain ganglia (collections of nerve cell bodies outside the central nervous system). How they do this remains unclear but may be related to the fact that neurons themselves do not reproduce.

Equally unclear is the relationship between this kind of latency and the long latent period between infection with HSV II and the development of cervical cancer (if the virus is indeed causative). According to Roizman, one possible hypothesis—but certainly not the only one—involves three steps: (i) The virus is maintained in a latent form in cells other than neurons (cervical epithelial cells, for example). (ii) When the virus is induced to multiply, defective virus is produced in addition to complete virus. (iii) The defective virus then transforms some cells, while cells infected by the complete virus die. Roizman points out that there is no evidence for the first of these steps, partial evidence for the second, and good evidence from Rapp's laboratory and his own for the third.

Finally, there is the possibility that two or more viruses may cooperate in initiating transformation. For example, Sol Spiegelman and his colleagues at Columbia University, New York City, found particles resembling RNA tumor viruses in Burkitt's lymphoma cells. These findings raised the possibility of an interaction between EBV and an oncogenic RNA virus in Burkitt's tumors. Spiegelman and his colleagues used an animal model to test this hypothesis. From experiments on chickens, in which they studied the interaction of Marek's disease virus (an oncogenic herpesvirus of chicken) and an RNA tumor virus, Spiegelman concluded that both could contribute to tumor growth under their experimental conditions.

Although evidence implicating DNA viruses in the etiology of human cancer is accumulating, numerous questions remain unanswered: What viral genes are necessary for transformation? Where and how is the virus maintained in the human body during the long latent period before cancer develops? How is viral DNA incorporated into cellular DNA? What controls the expression of viral DNA and triggers transformation? What is the role in cancer initiation of other human cancer virus candidates? of chemicals? and of the immune system? The cancer problem sometimes seems to have as many questions as Hydra has heads—and when one is lopped off, two grow back.

Identification of a viral role in the etiology of cancer could open the door to developing a vaccine to prevent the cancer. Carcinomas—the type of cancer associated with herpes simplex viruses—are by far the most common, accounting for some 85 percent of human cancer. A number of carcinomas, including those of the cervix and nasopharynx, are among the cancers linked to herpesviruses. An effective vaccine would thus be a major contribution to human welfare. The way to achieving this goal, however, is beset with even more perils and difficulties than are usually encountered in vaccine development.

A typical antiviral vaccine consists of a virus preparation that will elicit an immune response and enable the host to fight off subsequent invasion by the virus. The virus used for vaccination must be either inactivated or attenuated so that it cannot produce serious disease. Alternatively, it can be a relative of the pathogen which resembles it sufficiently to provoke an immune response but not enough to cause a severe infection. The cowpox virus used for smallpox vaccine is a good example of the latter.

A current example—and one relating directly to the cancer problem—is the vaccine developed for Marek's disease by B. R. Burmester, H. Graham Purchase, and their colleagues at the U.S. Department of Agriculture's Regional Poultry Research Laboratory in East Lansing, Michigan. Marek's disease is a malignant lymphoma of chickens. It is also an infectious disease caused by a herpesvirus, Marek's disease virus (MDV). For their vaccine, the East Lansing group used a herpesvirus of turkeys that is related immunologically to MDV but apparently not pathogenic to either species. Immunization with the turkey virus prevents Marek's disease but does not prevent reproduction of MDV (which occurs in the feather follicles) or virus spread.

The ability to induce lymphomas in primates with EBV and herpesvirus saimiri has provided models even more pertinent to the problem of human cancer. Recently, R. Laufs of the University of Göttingen, West Germany, used a vaccine prepared from killed herpesvirus saimiri to immunize cotton-topped marmosets against the lymphoma induced by that virus. The virus was killed by heating followed by treatment with formaldehyde. The vaccinated animals had high levels of antibodies to the virus in their blood. When challenged with massive doses of live herpesvirus saimiri, the immunized marmosets survived two to three times longer than did the control animals.

Use of a technique analogous to the one for the Marek's disease vaccine to produce a cancer vaccine for humans would be fraught with hazard, to say the least; it would be necessary to prove—somehow—that a relative of a human cancer virus candidate had no oncogenic potential in humans. Administration of an inactivated candidate virus may not solve the problem. Although Laufs found that his vaccine did not appear to induce cancer in immunized animals, Fred Rapp has shown that HSV I and HSV II, following photodynamic inactivation and loss of infectivity, still transformed hamster cells, as did HSV inactivated by ultraviolet light. Heat-inactivated viruses can also retain their oncogenic capacity, according to Dharam Ablashi and his colleagues. Herpesvirus saimiri, after heating to 56°C, could not infect and kill cultured cells, but it induced malignant lymphomas when injected into owl monkeys. In view of the theories that cancer is caused by defective DNA viruses, inactivation may actually increase the hazards.

Investigatiors are exploring approaches to vaccine development that do not require the injection of viral DNA—presumably carrying information necessary for transformation—into humans. Among them are the use of proteins or glycoproteins of the viral envelope or membrane or of virus-associated antigens from transformed cells to elicit an immune response in the host. Although these strategies avoid administration of genetic information to humans, they could be ineffective if the antigens are only weak stimulants of the immune system, or if the immune system is itself defective and cannot make an adequate response—a possibility considered by some to contribute to cancer initiation.

A final problem is the inadequacy of current techniques for assessing vaccine effectiveness. Onset of clinical symptoms cannot serve as a useful criterion. Most herpesvirus infections are not accompanied by detectable symptoms, and cancer itself has a long latent period between infection and disease development. Nor would the presence of circulating antibodies be indicative of vaccine effectiveness; recurrent infections can occur in individuals who have such antibodies. Additional information about the response of the immune system to herpesvirus infection will be required before suitable criteria for vaccine effectiveness can be selected.

Researchers are hopeful that they can develop a vaccine against human cancer, but these problems, plus the need for thorough testing for safety and effectiveness in animals before human studies can be initiated, all militate against an early solution.

4
RNA Viruses
The Age of Innocence Ends

Virologists have traditionally been among the most optimistic of cancer investigators, and for many of them the 1960's were an era of relative innocence. Secure in the knowledge that viruses cause tumors in animals, they were confident that these agents would provide an elegantly simple solution to the problem of human malignancies. If only a human cancer virus could be isolated, many virologists argued, a vaccine could be developed and control of cancer would be a reality.

That attitude engendered a tremendous outpouring of research results—a large number of little-recognized successes and a few more highly publicized failures. The investigators developed tissue culture systems for growing large numbers of virus particles, and thus learned a great deal about the biochemistry of oncogenic (tumor-forming) viruses. They discovered many animal tumor virus systems that served as models for what might occur in humans, and thus learned a great deal about the interaction of virus and host. They also isolated several putative human cancer viruses, and thus learned a great deal about humiliation and the loss of credibility as one after another of the ballyhooed candidates proved to be of nonhuman origin.

The age of innocence has slowly drawn to a close, however, as many virologists have begun to recognize that the problem is much more complex than they had anticipated. Although some still argue that a tangible oncogenic human virus will eventually be isolated, a growing number of investigators have concluded that this approach may be futile and have begun to reconsider the fundamental concepts of the nature of viruses and their role in animal biochemistry.

If viruses do play a causative role in human malignancies, these scientists suggest, it is most likely that the active agent is an incomplete or defective portion of one virus—or perhaps of several viruses—whose normal function is beneficial to the host. Research on oncogenic animal viruses, as a consequence, has been somewhat de-emphasized as investigators have pressed the search for virus fragments or information in human tumors. Nonetheless, there has been a continuing strong interest in ascertaining the normal role of oncogenic viruses, particularly those whose hereditary information is contained as RNA.

Oncogenic RNA viruses (also called oncornaviruses and RNA tumor viruses) are generally divided into three main classes, labeled A, B, and C. Type C RNA viruses, the most important class, have been shown to infect a large number of animal species. Most type C RNA viruses are oncogenic, causing mainly leukemias, lymphomas, and sarcomas—all tumors arising in tissues of mesodermal origin, such as bone, cartilage, connective tissue, and lymph nodes. Type B RNA viruses, which are fewer in number, have been associated primarily with certain tumors (carcinomas) of the breast. Type A RNA viruses, which are not infectious, are a very small group of viruslike particles that have not been found outside the confines of cells and that have not been shown to be oncogenic.

A principal difference between oncornaviruses and other animal RNA viruses lies in the size of the genome, the complete set of hereditary information contained in the chromosomes. Oncornavirus genomes have a mass of about 12×10^6 daltons, compared to about 6×10^6 daltons for the paramyxoviruses and about 2×10^6 daltons for poliomyelitis virus. Perhaps as a result of this large genome, oncornaviruses have a more complex internal structure with no clearly observable symmetry. They may also contain more types of proteins and more species of nucleic acids.

Distinctions among the various types of oncornaviruses have been based on morphology, but they can also be made on immunological differences and modes of maturation. The type C RNA viruses consist of a roughly spherical, compact nucleoid (that is, RNA and the associated proteins) surrounded by an electron-lucent lipid layer that gives electron micrographs of the virus a targetlike appearance (Figure 8E). The nucleoid of the type B viruses is more eccentric in shape (Figure 8D), apparently because its major internal protein is about two-thirds larger than that of the type C viruses. The glycoprotein surface spikes of the type B viruses are also larger and more regularly spaced than those of the type C viruses.

The type A particles occur in two subtypes, one found in cellular cytoplasm and one found in cisternae, reservoirs for lymph and other body fluids. Those found in the cytoplasm are believed to be immature forms of type B viruses, to which they are immunologically similar, and there is speculation that those in the cisternae are immature type C particles. The morphology of type A particles is similar to that of the other viruses (Figure 8A), but the type A particles are encapsulated by a protein shell rather than by a lipid-containing membrane.

The most important characteristic of the oncornaviruses is that they contain an RNA-directed DNA polymerase, or reverse transcriptase. Reverse transcriptase was discovered in 1970 by Howard M. Temin and Satoshi Mizutani of the McArdle Laboratory for Cancer Research at the University of Wisconsin Medical School, Madison, and independently by David Baltimore of the Massachusetts Institute of Technology, Cambridge. Discovery of this enzyme, which mediates the synthesis of DNA from an RNA template, provided the first biochemical evidence of a mechanism for perpetuation of the viral genome when a cell divides.

After an oncornavirus has entered a cell and shed its protein coat, the first important step in infection, most investigators now agree, is production of a DNA copy of the viral genome by the reverse transcriptase. Several lines of evidence confirm the presence of this intermediate, called the provirus, but perhaps the most conclusive evidence is provided by M. Hill and Jana Hillova of the Institut Gustave-Roussy in Villejuif, France. They found that RNA-free DNA from chicken cells transformed by Rous sarcoma virus in turn transforms uninfected chicken cells and mediates the production of more Rous virus. H. Hanafusa of the Public Health Research Institute of the City of New York has also shown that mutant type C RNA viruses that do not contain a reverse transcriptase are not infectious.

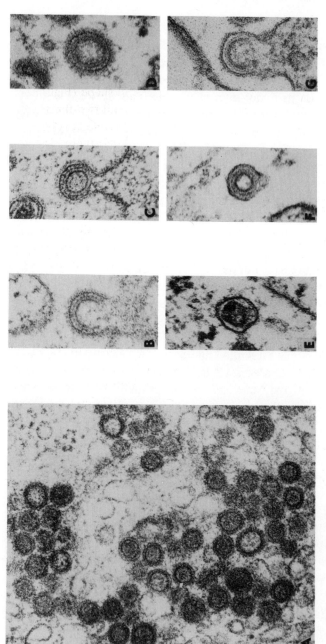

FIGURE 8. Electron micrographs of oncornaviruses [magnifications: (A) ~ ×100,000; (B to G) ~ ×140,000]. (A) Group of intracytoplasmic type A particles in a mouse mammary tumor. (B) Type B particle budding from a mouse mammary tumor cell. (C) Late bud of type B particle from mouse mammary tumor. (D) Free, immature, type B particle with spikes on surface, electron–lucent center in the nucleoid, and spokes radiating from outer surface of the nucleoid to inner surface of the envelope. (E) Type C particle in extracellular space (F) Late bud of type C particle in tissue of human embryo kidney cells infected with a strain of Rauscher leukemia virus. (G) Type C particle budding from human embryo lung cell in tissue culture infected with feline leukemia virus. [Source: Albert J. Dalton, National Cancer Institute].

The provirus, once formed, is generally believed to be integrated into the host cell's genome to produce a virogene—a gene that is the template for the production of a virus. (The terms provirus and virogene are often considered synonymous.) Several investigators have shown that the virus contains an endonuclease, an exonuclease, and a ligase, all the enzymes necessary for cleaving cellular DNA, inserting the provirus, and mending the break. There is no evidence that these enzymes actually perform this function.

Once the provirus is integrated, several alternative pathways are possible. Since the host's immune systems react primarily to viral proteins, integration provides a way for the provirus to replicate while remaining shielded from the immune defenses. Proliferation of the infected cell results in transmission of the virogene to the daughter cells without the appearance of viral protein or intact viruses. If the infected cell is a germ cell, moreover, the virogene is also transmitted to the host's progeny. Parental infection of progeny is known as vertical transmission.

Under certain, as yet undetermined circumstances, the virogene can be activated, and the cell will begin producing new virus particles that may infect neighboring cells or other organisms of the same species. This type of transmission is known as horizontal transmission. And finally, if the virus is oncogenic or if it acquires additional information to become oncogenic, the same set of circumstances that initiate virus production—or perhaps a slightly different set of circumstances that activate only part of the virogene—may convert the infected cell into a tumor cell.

This last possibility, which is one manifestation of the oncogene theory developed by Robert J. Huebner and George J. Todaro of the National Cancer Institute (NCI) in Bethesda, Maryland, is still considered rather speculative. But the other alternatives are supported by firm experimental evidence, the foremost of which is the induction of type C RNA viruses from apparently virus-free cells.

This induction was first demonstrated in 1971 by Wallace P. Rowe of the National Institute of Allergy and Infectious Diseases, Bethesda, Maryland. Rowe cultured cells from a strain of mice with a high natural incidence of leukemia and exposed the cells to certain types of chemical mutagens such as bromodeoxyuridine. After this exposure, the cells began to produce an RNA virus similar to, but distinct from, the murine leukemia virus. Subsequent experiments by several others have shown that such viruses, called endogenous viruses, can be induced in many cell lines, including cells from animals with a low natural incidence of tumors. None of the endogenous viruses induced in this fashion have been shown to be oncogenic, however.

More recently, Robert M. McAllister of the University of Southern California Medical School, Los Angeles, inadvertently discovered an apparently different type of endogenous virus. McAllister injected cells from a human sarcoma into the brain of a kitten and observed the release of a type C RNA virus, called RD-114, that he initially thought might be a human cancer virus. Intensive investigations in his and a half-dozen other laboratories, however, soon revealed that RD-114 was actually a hitherto unknown feline RNA virus distinct from the well-known feline leukemia virus.

Unlike the chemically induced viruses, which replicate to a limited extent in the species of origin, RD-114 will not, in general, replicate in feline cells. It was thus one of the first examples of a class now known as xenotropic viruses—endogenous viruses that do not, under most conditions, replicate in the species of origin. It is possible that the chemically induced viruses are merely forms of the xenotropic viruses that have mutated slightly so that they can replicate in the species of origin, but there is no firm evidence to support this thesis.

Xenotropic viruses have also been isolated from several other species, including chickens, hamsters, mice, rats, and pigs. It now seems possible, moreover, that each species has a unique virus shared by all its members. Jay A. Levy of the Cancer Research Institute at the University of California, San Francisco, has demonstrated, for example, that apparently identical xenotropic viruses can be isolated from all strains of mice, including wild field mice, that he has examined. The limited evidence yet available suggests that an analogous situation occurs in other species.

There are apparent exceptions to the principle that xenotropic viruses will not grow in the species of origin. Many investigators have observed what they thought to be type C RNA viruses in tissues from a variety of species, but have assumed that the viruses were not infectious because they did not proliferate in cultures of the same tissues. These observations have occurred most frequently in embryonic and placental tissues.

S. S. Kalter and his associates at the Southwest Foundation for Research and Education, San Antonio, Texas, have obtained electron micrographs of what appear to be endogenous type C particles in baboon and monkey placentas. These putative viruses do not replicate in cultured primate placental cells, but Todaro has shown that those from the baboon will infect dog brain tissues, and several investigators are now attempting to characterize them. Kalter and others have also observed such particles in human placental tissue, but no one has yet been able to find tissues in which these putative endogenous human viruses will replicate. None of the xenotropic viruses have been shown to be oncogenic in any species.

The scenario that has emerged from these findings is thus considerably more complicated—and confusing—than that which was envisioned only 2 or 3 years ago. Whereas virologists were then fairly confident that one virus might be the cause of any particular tumor, they are now faced with the possibility that two, three, or perhaps even more might be involved.

At least one strain of mice, Huebner points out, is already known to harbor three different type C RNA viruses. The first, believed to be an exogenous virus, is the principal virus isolated from mouse tumors (murine leukemia virus) and produces tumors when injected into newborn mice of the same strain. The second, a chemically induced endogenous virus, replicates poorly in embryonic mouse cells in culture and does not produce tumors in newborn mice. The third, also an endogenous virus, does not replicate in cultured mouse cells and does not produce tumors. Even though the last two types do not produce tumors in newborn mice, many virologists think that these types are nonetheless implicated in the etiology of cancer. There is some evidence to suggest that a similar number of RNA viruses may occur in animals of other species, but the extrapolation to humans is still speculative since there is as yet no firm evidence for the presence of complete type C RNA viruses in human tumors.

The situation becomes even more complicated when DNA viruses are brought into the picture. Sol Spiegelman and his associates at Columbia University's Institute for Cancer Research, New York City, have reported that the incidence of Marek's disease, a lymphoma of chickens, increases in fowls exposed to both a DNA virus (Marek's disease herpesvirus) and a type C RNA virus called Rous associated virus type 2. Chickens are also known to have a virogene that can produce at least one endogenous virus that may be implicated in the etiology of Marek's disease.

An even more complex situation is observed in human nasopharyngeal carcinoma, a malignancy of the nasal cavity, pharynx, and oral cavity. By molecular hybridization, Harald Zur-Hausen of the University of Erlangen-Nuremberg, Erlangen, West Germany, has found in nasopharyngeal tumors DNA sequences homologous to those of the Epstein-Barr virus, a DNA herpesvirus that has been tentatively associated with some types of cancer. This finding suggests that the virus—or hereditary information derived from it—is involved in the etiology of the tumor.

Spiegelman, using a similar technique, has reported that nasopharyngeal tumors contain DNA sequences homologous to RNA sequences in a type C RNA virus that causes similar tumors in experimental animals. And Albert Sabin, while working at NCI's Frederick Cancer Research Center in Frederick, Maryland, has reported that the tumors contain an antigen (a protein or glycoprotein that elicits an immune response) characteristic of the herpes simplex virus. Many virologists also believe, as is suggested by the observation of placental particles, that humans have a virogene that can produce at least one type C RNA virus. There are, then, four types of viruses that might be associated with this tumor.

Most of the evidence suggesting this complexity has been developed within the last year, and the investigators have had little time to sort out all of the implications. But the steady accretion of unexpected new results has initiated a major rethinking of the nature of viruses and of their role in the transmission of hereditary information within and between organisms.

In the first place, many investigators are beginning to accept the conclusion that infectious oncogenic viruses are the exception rather than the rule. Strongly transforming viruses such as the Rous sarcoma virus, which transforms nearly all the cells it infects, are very rare. They can be maintained only by passage through laboratory animals, and are generally agreed to be artifacts.

Those oncornaviruses that do cause tumors in nonlaboratory animals are only weakly transforming. These viruses are generally transmitted from parent to progeny, but some have been shown to be infectious also. William Hardy and Lloyd Old of the Memorial Sloan-Kettering Cancer Center in New York City recently demonstrated, for example, that feline leukemia virus is transmitted both vertically and horizontally.

In most cases, tumors are a very rare response to infection by oncornaviruses; their efficiencies of transformation are as much as a dozen powers of 10 lower than that of the Rous sarcoma virus. When transformation does occur, moreover, the responsible virus can generally be recovered from the tumor or its presence can be demonstrated in some other manner. Since such viruses have never been definitively demonstrated in human tumors, Temin reasons, it seems likely that the oncogenic animal viruses provide an analogy for human cancers rather than an etiology. That is, experiments with the oncornaviruses are useful in providing information about the formation and expression of genes that might be responsible for malignancies in humans, but it is unlikely that an infectious virus causes cancer in humans.

One of the major conclusions that some scientists have reached from animal experiments is that a virus must be integrated into the host cell's genome before it can transform the cell. A corollary to this conclusion is that transformation is controlled genetically rather than epigenetically; that is, transformation can be caused only by a change in gene structure and not by cellular changes altering gene expression. Many scientists, particularly some of those investigating chemical carcinogenesis, would disagree with this latter conclusion.

But whether the mechanism is genetic or epigenetic, all the evidence indicates that only RNA viruses that contain a reverse transcriptase are potentially oncogenic. (DNA viruses, of course, can be integrated directly and thus do not exhibit this requirement.) Neither the presence of a reverse transcriptase nor integration, however, is sufficient for oncogenicity. Todaro and Wade Parks of NCI have suggested, for example, that syncytium-forming RNA viruses (viruses that cause cells to fuse into large masses) replicate through a DNA intermediate but are not oncogenic, possibly because they replicate in the cell's cytoplasm and are thus physically separated from the cellular DNA. And Harold E. Varmus of the University of California, San Francisco, and Ashley Haase of the San Francisco Veteran's Administration Hospital have shown that visna virus—a sheep virus which has never been demonstrated to cause tumors in animals—replicates through an integrated DNA intermediate.

If it is granted, then, that oncogenic information must be integrated in the host genome at the time of tumorigenesis, there are two main theories about how the information gets there if there is no exogenous infection. The oncogene theory (Figure 9), proposed by Huebner and Todaro in 1969, postulates that the virogene, which is now thought to be present in all cells, contains oncogenic information that is normally repressed by cellular mechanisms. The virogene, according to this theory, thus contains an oncogene, a segment of the genome that contains information necessary for the transformation of cells.

/ The protovirus theory, proposed by Temin in 1970, postulates that the virogene or a precursor is, in effect, highly mutable, and that oncogenic information is occasionally synthesized de novo. The

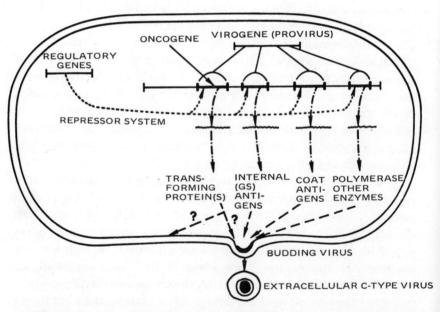

FIGURE 9. The oncogene hypothesis postulates that tumors are induced by transforming proteins which are coded for by an oncogene. The oncogene is part of a larger structure, a virogene, which has the capacity to produce a complete tumor virus. Theoretically, oncogenes are turned off in normal cells by regulatory genes that code for a repressor system. [Source: Robert J. Huebner, National Cancer Institute]

oncogene theory thus predicts that information for transformation is transmitted vertically through the germ line, whereas the protovirus theory predicts that only the potential for synthesis of the information is transmitted/Neither theory requires the expression of complete virus particles for the initiation of cancer.

The oncogene theory represented a significant extrapolation from existing data. In one sense, however, it might be termed an ad hoc theory: It provides a possible explanation for tumorigenesis, but it offers no normal role for the oncogene or the virogene. In the absence of a normal role, many scientists argue, there would be no evolutionary pressure for maintenance of the gene—it would provide no benefit or advantage to the host organism—and it is unlikely that it would be universally incorporated in animals, as the virogene appears to be.

The oncogene theory also predicts a relatively static genome, whereas much recent evidence suggests that the interaction between virus and genome produces a great deal of change. The oncogene theory is thus falling into disfavor among virologists, although not all who reject it would embrace the protovirus theory.

The protovirus theory, on the contrary, offers a method by which genetic evolution can occur in cells other than germ cells. Temin suggests that the normal function of the virogene is to provide information transfer between cells or between chromosomes in one cell, and perhaps to provide for the synthesis of new hereditary information. The synthesis of genetic information necessary for oncogenesis could thus be simply a normal—albeit rare—result of the functioning of this system.

In simplest terms, the protovirus theory suggests that the protovirus (virogene) directs the production of an RNA copy of certain segments of the cellular genome and then packages the copy and a reverse transcriptase in a form that is able to enter the nucleus of a neighboring cell. In the infected cell, the reverse transcriptase produces a DNA copy of the RNA, which is integrated into that cell's genome. This process may also occur at a different site on the genome of the original cell.

After integration, the new information may simply remain quiescent in the host's genome, it may alter the biochemistry of the host cell, or it may be repackaged to infect other cells, depending on the state of the host cell's genetic controls. This transfer of information from DNA to RNA to DNA could serve, for example, to recruit and identify cells during the process of embryonic induction (differentiation) and to permit new genetic information to be encoded during the lifetime of a single organism (gene amplification).

The possibility for generation of new information arises if either the transcription, the integration, or both, are not precise. Consider, for illustration, the hypothetical sequences *abcdefgh* in the genome of one cell and *lmnopqrs* in that of another, and suppose that normal functioning of the virogene would involve transcription of *abcd* from the first and insertion of this fragment between *m* and *n* in the second. If a mistake were made in transcription, the resultant sequence in the second cell might be *lmbcdenopqrs*.

Most of the time, this newly synthesized information (*mb* and *en*) will be either nonsense or irrelevant to the cell, and in some cases perhaps even lethal. But in a small number of cases, the new information will be beneficial to the host organism, and in even a smaller number of cases, the new information may be oncogenic. If the protovirus does not integrate at a predetermined site, this process might also lead to a random selection and interchange of genes; development of the potential for transformation might then simply require the side-by-side alignment of preexisting genes (Figure 10) without a requirement for synthesis of new information. In either case, once the oncogenic information is present in the cell, transformation can occur without the expression of viral particles.

An analogous type of process has been demonstrated for DNA viruses that integrate into the cellular genome. That process is somewhat different, however, in that the DNA which forms the new virus is physically excised from the cellular genome. Imprecise excision can thus leave some of the viral DNA behind and incorporate host DNA into the new virus. Ernst Winocur and Niza Frankel of the Weizmann Institute in Israel have shown, for example, that polyoma and SV40 viruses contain increasingly greater amounts of host DNA after serial passage through cultured cells. After six passages, they find, as much as 50 percent of the DNA in the virus is of host origin.

There is much less data to support this possibility for RNA viruses (Figure 11). One important requirement of the protovirus theory is that a reverse transcriptase must be present in healthy cells, and this requirement has been a major stumbling block. Several early reports of reverse transcriptases in normal cells have subsequently been discounted because

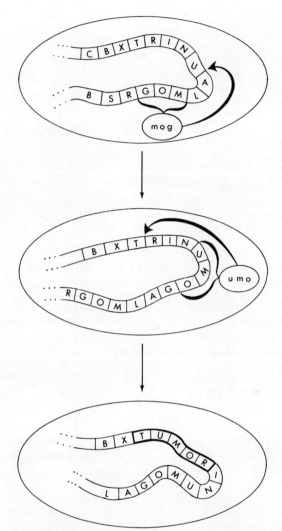

FIGURE 10. One method by which the protovirus
can realign chromosomes within a cell to produce
oncogenic information. The protovirus transcribes a
segment of the gene into RNA (lowercase letters),
which is then copied into DNA and inserted into the
chromosome at a new location. Repetition of this
process can, in some cases, produce a side-by-side
alignment of the genes (outlined in bold) that are
necessary for carcinogenesis.

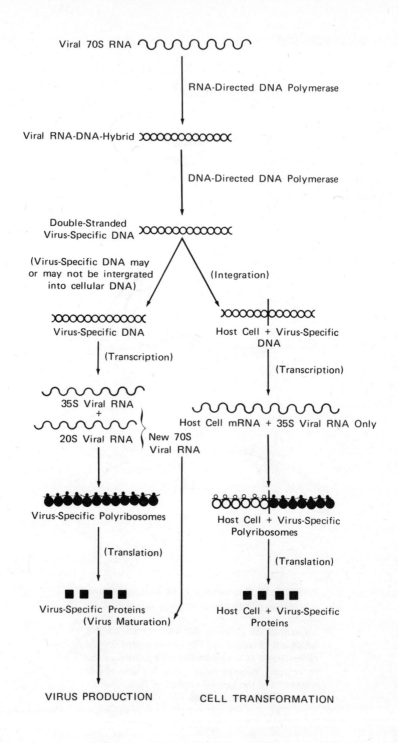

they were based on results obtained with a synthetic RNA template that has since been shown to be nonspecific for reverse transcriptase. Only Temin has thus far been able to demonstrate conclusively that this situation does occur.

In 1972, Temin and Chil-Yong Kang of the McArdle Laboratory reported reverse transcriptase activity in uninfected chicken embryos and demonstrated that the responsible enzyme is distinct from the reverse transcriptases in avian oncornaviruses. Unlike viral reverse transcriptase, however, the chick embryo enzyme does not accept exogenous RNA as a template, indicating that it has great specificity for a particular cellular RNA. Robert C. Gallo of NCI has produced less definitive evidence suggesting that a similar reverse transcriptase activity may be present in normal human lymphocytes. (This activity, however, is observed only when the lymphocytes are treated with phytohemagglutinin, a chemical that stimulates mitosis.) These reports have provided the first major evidence in support of the protovirus theory.

Temin has, in fact, carried the protovirus theory one step further. Last year, he and Mizutani demonstrated that the reverse transcriptase of a new avian oncornavirus, reticuloendotheliosis virus, is closely related serologically to the normal chick embryo DNA polymerase and to the reverse transcriptases of other avian oncornaviruses (which are less closely related to the normal polymerase). It is quite possible then, that the reverse transcriptase in reticuloendotheliosis virus has evolved from the normal cellular polymerase, and that the other avian reverse transcriptases have also evolved from this source. Gallo has observed the same type of relationship between a human DNA polymerase and reverse transcriptases from primate oncornaviruses.

Temin thus suggests that the avian oncornaviruses, and perhaps all oncornaviruses, have evolved from normal cellular components. At some point in history, conceivably, the endogenous viruses have mutated in such a fashion that they were freed from the cell's genetic controls and became able to replicate in other cells. The major evolutionary changes, Gallo adds, may have occurred when the viruses crossed interspecies barriers.

FIGURE 11. Virus replication and cell transformation by RNA tumor viruses. See text for details. [Source: William M. Shannon, Southern Research Institute, Birmingham, Alabama].

The implication, then, is that genetic controls are more effective in humans than in other species, or perhaps evolutionary pressures are different, so that endogenous human viruses have not been able to escape from cellular control. Although endogenous human viruses may be able to assemble or synthesize oncogenic information in susceptible cells, the virus that has done the assembling has not yet been able to escape and infect other humans.

The cancer virologists have thus gotten results substantially different than those they had originally bargained for. The situation is, in fact, quite analogous to that immediately after World War II when physicists naively set out to build a fusion power plant and instead created the new discipline of plasma physics. The virologists set out to isolate a human cancer virus and instead appear to have created a new discipline of (for lack of a better term) viral genetics.

5
Tumor Immunology
The Host's Response to Cancer

No one worries about the growth of cancer cells in culture systems or in test tubes. Only when they grow in the living—human—organism is there cause for alarm. Culture systems are valuable for studying the basic mechanisms of oncogenesis, but it is the response of the whole individual to his disease that is of prime importance because this interaction between host and disease determines the patient's prognosis. Many investigators think that the immune system is a major component of an individual's response to cancer. They are now seeking the answers to two questions of fundamental importance: What is the role played by the immune system in the initiation and growth of tumors? And, how may the immune system be manipulated to cure or control cancers in humans?

Since deficiencies in the immune responses of cancer patients are well documented, there is little doubt that the immune system is somehow involved in oncogenesis. The uncertainty concerns its role—whether the deficiencies are the cause or effect of the disease and whether the immune system hinders or promotes tumor growth. Determining the nature of immune system involvement in cancer development is thus critically important for devising strategies for immunotherapy.

Immunotherapy—the manipulation of immune responses for cancer treatment—is considered by some investigators to hold the greatest promise for a cancer cure. Techniques employing surgery and radiation are restricted in application. They can eliminate the primary cancer but are of little value in controlling metastasis, the spread of cancer throughout the body. Chemotherapy, which aims to kill all cancer cells regardless of their location, has proved successful in controlling certain kinds of relatively rare cancers, like Hodgkin's disease and some leukemias, but not more common cancers, like those of the lung and colon. Consequently, many investigators are turning to immunotherapeutic techniques. Some of their early clinical trials—and they emphasize the preliminary, experimental nature of the studies—have produced results that have encouraged them to proceed, but with caution.

The caution stems from observations that in some studies with animals, and possibly with humans, stimulation of the immune system produced enhancement, not inhibition, of tumor growth. Complexity appears to be the rule for cancer research, and tumor immunology is no exception. Immune responses require a number of components, including several different cell types and an assortment of factors, which may or may not interact with one another. Thus, despite recent progress, immune response mechanisms are incompletely understood, and there is still uncertainty about how they can best be manipulated for the cancer patient's benefit.

The early history of tumor immunology research was inauspicious. Investigations at the beginning of this century purported to show that animals immunized with material prepared from a transplantable tumor resisted tumor growth when they were subsequently challenged with live tumor cells. The tumor cells grew and formed tumors in nonimmunized animals. The experiments suffered from a major flaw, however: At that time, there were no inbred strains of animals. Resistance to the tumor challenge was due, not to recognition and rejection of specific tumor antigens, but to an immune response directed against normal tissue antigens from a genetically dissimilar animal.

All cells carry genetically determined antigens. (Antigens are any substances that stimulate an immune response; most are chemically complex materials like proteins or nucleic acids.) An individual does not normally mount an immune attack on antigens of his own tissues, but cells with different antigens from another individual are recognized as foreign and attacked by the immune system. Identical twins can tolerate each other's cells because they are genetically the same. This is also true for members of the same inbred strain of laboratory animals, which have very similar, if not indentical, genetic compositions. Development and use of these strains has greatly facilitated immunological research.

Scientists now think that most (but not all) tumor cells carry membrane antigens called tumor-associated antigens that do differ from those of the host's normal cells. Proving that these antigens are absolutely tumor-specific (found only in tumors and not in normal cells at any time during development) is extremely difficult and remains a major problem of tumor immunology. Investigators have established, in both in vivo and in vitro systems, that animals can mount an immune response against tumor cells. For example, after a chemically induced tumor is surgically removed from a mouse, the animal can resist tumor growth when viable cells of that same tumor are injected. It cannot resist the growth of a tumor induced by another chemical and carrying antigens different from those of the first tumor. These experiments demonstrate that when an animal has once been exposed to tumor antigens they can be recognized on subsequent exposure and tumor growth resisted; that is, the animal can be immunized against the tumor. In addition, numerous investigators have shown that effector cells ("killer" cells or small lymphocytes) of the immune system can recognize and destroy cultured tumor cells.

Both of these concepts—tumor-associated antigenicity and the capacity of the host to make an effective immune response to tumor antigens—underlie the theory of immunological surveillance now favored by a majority of tumor immunologists. According to this theory, tumor cells constantly arise in complex organisms such as man, but because of their "foreignness," they are efficiently eliminated by the immune system of most individuals. Occasionally, however, tumor cells escape the immune system's surveillance. They can then proliferate—and cancer results.

Evidence supporting the immune surveillance theory includes observations that the cancer incidence is higher in people with less effective immune systems than in those with strong responses. The immune system is thought to deteriorate with increasing age, and the incidence of cancer is known to be higher in the elderly. Cancer afflicts up to 10 percent of patients with certain genetic immunodeficiency diseases, according to Robert Good of Memorial Sloan-Kettering Cancer Center, New York City, Thomas Waldman of the National Cancer Institute (NCI),

Bethesda, Maryland, and others who have investigated these diseases. Since many of these patients are young, their cancer incidence is far higher than that of normal individuals of the same age.

Patients who have undergone immunosuppressive therapy for the treatment of disease—including cancer—or to prevent rejection of organ transplants are also prone to a higher cancer incidence. Israel Penn and his colleagues at the University of Colorado, Denver, found that patients with kidney transplants had an incidence of cancer approximately 100 times greater than that of the general population in the same age range. The chemicals used for treating cancer also suppress immune responses. These observations have led to the suggestion that intermittent chemotherapeutic regimes that allow recovery of the patient's immune response may be more beneficial to the patient than continuous administration of the drugs.

Graft or transplant rejection and tumor surveillance are thought to be effected by the same components of the immune system. The immune system consists of two major functional branches—cell-mediated and humoral immunity. Cell-mediated immunity is the province of T or thymus-dependent lymphycytes (Figure 12A) that act directly to destroy foreign antigens. They are involved in transplant rejection and immune surveillance, and also in delayed hypersensitivity reactions and resistance to viral infections. An example of a delayed hypersensitivity reaction is the skin response of redness and swelling that may occur 24 to 48 hours after antigens are injected subcutaneously. Such skin tests are frequently employed to assess the immunocompetence (the ability to respond to antigens) of cancer patients.

Humoral immunity depends on the production of soluble antibodies by plasma cells. Plasma cells differentiate from B (for bone marrow) lymphocytes (Figure 12B) when they are stimulated by an antigen. Antibodies circulate in the blood and are required for resistance to a number of bacterial infections. They combine with antigens and make them more susceptible to destruction.

Needless to say, the situation is more complex than indicated by this brief explanation. The two branches of the immune system interact in a manner not completely understood at present. Numerous factors elaborated by lymphoid cells also participate in the responses. In addition, a third cell type, the macrophage, may be important for tumor cell

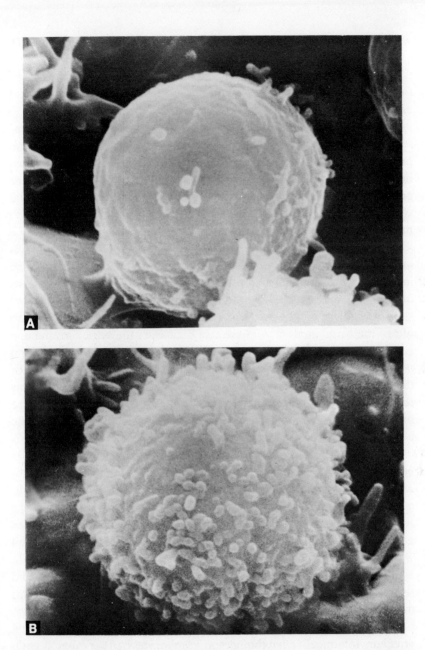

FIGURE 12. Scanning electron micrographs of a T lymphocyte (A) and a B lymphocyte (B). The surfaces of the two cells are distinctly different—B cells have a large number of fingerlike projections (called villi) and T cells have a relatively smooth surface. [Source: Memorial Sloan-Kettering Cancer Center and Rockefeller University]

destruction. Macrophages are large mobile cells, produced by the organs (including the liver and spleen) of the reticuloendothelial system, that can engulf and destroy particulate matter, including other cells.

If the immune surveillance theory is assumed to be correct, researchers must then explain how cancer cells can escape surveillance and produce tumors in normal people, that is, in people with no known immune deficiencies. A number of theories have been proposed. They need not be mutually exclusive; a system as complex as the immune system might malfunction in several different ways, each of which leads to the same result—tumor growth.

One escape mechanism thought to play a role in oncogenesis involves the presence of blocking factors in the blood serums of individuals with tumors. Ingegerd Hellström and Karl Erik Hellström of the University of Washington School of Medicine, Seattle, proposed this mechanism on the basis of results obtained with in vitro assays of cell-mediated immunity. These assays measure the cytotoxic effects— cell destruction or inhibition of cell division—of lymphocytes on target cells in culture. In order for lymphocytes to exert their cytotoxic effects, they must first be sensitized to antigens present on the target cells. This requires prior exposure, either in vivo or in vitro, of the lymphocytes to tumor cell antigens. Such sensitized lymphocytes are also called immune lymphocytes.

The Hellströms showed that lymphocytes taken from mice with growing sarcomas that had been induced with Moloney sarcoma virus were cytotoxic to Moloney sarcoma cells in culture. If the sarcoma cells were incubated with serum from animals with growing tumors before the lymphocytes were added (the serum was removed before lymphocyte addition), the lymphocytes no longer attacked the tumor cells. Incubation with serums from normal animals or animals with tumors unrelated to Moloney sarcoma had no effect on lymphocyte cytotoxicity. Neither did serum from animals whose tumors had regressed. The Hellströms interpreted these results as showing that mice with growing tumors produced "blocking factors" that prevented their lymphocytes from attacking tumor cells even though the lymphocytes had the capacity to do so. Blocking activity has since been detected in serums from several animal species with different tumors and also in serums from human cancer patients (Figure 13).

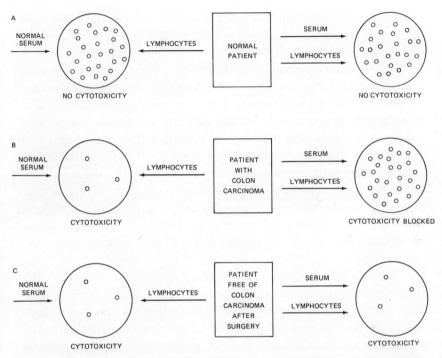

FIGURE 13. Schematic representation of the blocking phenomenon. (A) Colon carcinoma cells, growing in culture, are not recognized and destroyed by lymphocytes from a normal individual and continue to proliferate. (B) Lymphocytes taken before surgery from the patient who was the source of the tumor cells can destroy the cultured carcinoma cells that had been previously incubated with normal serum but not those incubated with the patient's own serum; this is blocking. (C) After surgery, when the patient is clinically free of tumor, his serum no longer exhibits blocking activity. [Source: Adapted from a diagram by Ingegerd Hellström and Karl Erik Hellström, University of Washington Medical School, Seattle]

Whenever in vitro assays are used, there is always the problem of whether the results are truly applicable to the situation in vivo. Here the question is whether the blocking activity demonstrated in vitro enables tumor cells to escape from immune surveillance in vivo. A number of investigators, including S. C. Bansal of the Medical College of Pennsylvania in Philadelphia and H. O. Sjögren of the University of Lund, Sweden, have shown that serums that block the cytotoxic activity of lymphocytes on cultured tumor cells also enhance the growth of tumors of the corresponding type that have been transplanted into animals.

Additional evidence for the importance of blocking factors in cancer etiology has been obtained by the Hellströms. They found that patients with primary melanoma that had not metastasized no longer had blocking activity in their serum after their tumors were removed surgically. Patients with progressive metastatic melanoma did have the activity. Finally, in patients who had been in remission from the disease and subsequently relapsed, blocking factor reappeared in the serum 2 to 6 months before their relapses were clinically detectable. Although these and other studies indicate that blocking factors may play a role in promoting or permitting tumor growth in vivo, the case has not yet been definitively proved. At the very least, however, knowledge of an individual's blocking factor status may be of diagnostic or prognostic value.

The biochemical nature of blocking factor is still uncertain. The Hellströms originally thought that it was antibody against tumor antigens. Such antibody could block by binding to antigen on tumor cell membranes and preventing attack by sensitized lymphocytes. If this were true, stimulation of the immune system as an immunotherapeutic strategy could do more harm than good if humoral immunity—and thus the production of blocking antibody—were stimulated in addition to cell-mediated immunity.

More recent evidence supports the hypothesis that blocking factor is either a complex of antibody with tumor antigen or is tumor antigen itself. The Hellströms, with Sjögren and Bansal, found that they could separate blocking factor into two fractions. One contained components, including antibodies, with molecular weights greater than 100,000; the other contained substances with lower molecular weights and included antigens. Under the standard conditions employed by the Hellströms for their in vitro assay system (incubation of cultured tumor cells with the material to be tested for blocking activity and removal of that material before addition of lymphocytes), both fractions were required for blocking activity. Antigen alone prevented the cytotoxic effects of lymphocytes but only when it remained with the lymphycytes throughout the entire test. Antigen may act directly on the lymphocytes rather than on the tumor cells.

Robert Baldwin and his associates at the University of Nottingham, England, have additional evidence that complexes of tumor antigens with antibody cause blocking. They isolated tumor-associated antigens from hepatoma cells. (A hepatoma is a liver tumor.) Serum taken from rats following surgical removal of their hepatomas contains antibody against tumor antigens but it does not block the cytotoxic effect of lymphocytes on cultured hepatoma cells. Baldwin and his colleagues could restore blocking activity by adding isolated antigen to the serum. Blocking occurred only when the proper ratio of antigen to antibody was attained. Addition of either too little or too much antigen to the serum produced no blocking activity. Baldwin thinks that large complexes of antibody with antigen, which can bind to tumor cells through the antibody moiety, block the access of lymphocytes to tumor cells more effectively than does antibody alone. Alternatively, the antigen portion may have a specific role in preventing lymphocyte activity on tumor cells.

In addition to blocking factor, the set of factors involved in tumor immunology includes unblocking factor. According to the Hellströms' definition, "unblocking" simply means that one serum can abrogate the blocking activity of another. For example, serum taken from mice whose Moloney sarcomas have spontaneously regressed nullifies the blocking activity of serum from mice with growing tumors. Baldwin obtained similar results using serum from mice whose hepatomas had been excised and serum from mice with growing tumors. Although the evidence is not yet conclusive, unblocking factor may be free antibody. This would be consistent with Baldwin's finding that blocking does not occur in the presence of excess free antibody.

Other investigators, including Graham Currie of the Chester Beatty Institute in London and Charles McKhann of the University of Minnesota Medical School, Minneapolis, have focused on the role of tumor antigens in oncogenesis. McKhann points out that tumors may have evolved the capacity to shed large quantities of antigen as a defense mechanism against immune surveillance. McKhann and Currie think that antigens shed by tumor cells permit tumor growth by binding to receptors on lymphocytes and preventing them from attacking tumor cells (Figure 14). Antigen could thus inhibit immune surveillance by binding directly to lymphocytes or by forming blocking complexes with antibody, or both. The effect would be to saturate and overwhelm the immune response.

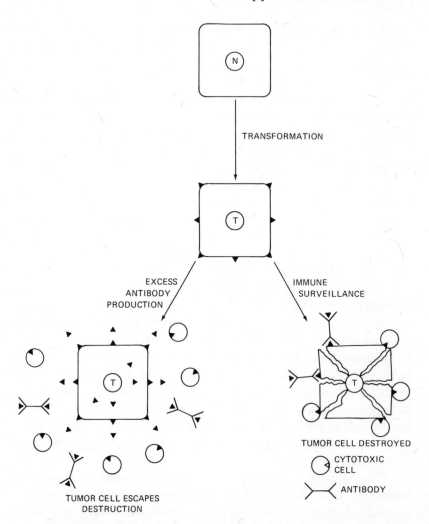

FIGURE 14. Transformation of a normal cell to a tumor cell results in expression of new tumor antigens (represented by the dark triangles) on the surface of the transformed cell. When immune surveillance is functioning properly, these antigens are recognized by antibodies and cytotoxic cells of the immune system that combine with the antigens on the cell surface and destroy the aberrant cell. If the cell sheds a large excess of antigen, however, the binding sites on the antibodies and cytotoxic cells will become saturated with it and unable to bind to the cell-surface antigens. [Source: Adapted from a diagram by Charles F. McKhann, University of Minnesota Medical School, Minneapolis]

This suggestion is consistent with observations that animals that have been immunized against a particular tumor can resist challenges with small doses of tumor cells but not with large ones. The immune system apparently does have a limit to its capacity to respond to antigens.

Pinning down the roles of antigen and antibody in tumor growth should facilitate rational design of immunotherapeutic approaches. Strategies to remove antigen by increasing its breakdown or to prevent its release from tumor cells might be feasible. So might strategies to increase cell-mediated or even humoral immunity.

One of the few investigators to challenge the current view of immune surveillance is Richmond Prehn of the Fox Chase Center for Cancer and Medical Sciences, Philadelphia, Pennsylvania. According to Prehn, weak immune responses, such as those that might occur in the initial stages of tumor growth when only a few aberrant cells are present, stimulate tumor growth rather than inhibiting it. The immune system does function as a defense against cancer, but, in Prehn's view, it acts too late and too inefficiently to be of much value for surveillance. He does think, however, that stimulating the immune system could still be useful for cancer therapy.

Prehn contends that there are alternate interpretations, consistent with his theory of immunostimulation of oncogenesis, that can be made of data already cited as evidence in favor of immune surveillance. For example, 50 percent or more of the cancers found in patients with immunodeficiency diseases or undergoing immunosuppressive treatments are leukemias, lymphomas, or other tumors of the lymphoreticular system. Immunosuppression and immune deficiency diseases directly affect this system. Thus, the increased malignancies may result from intrinsic or induced abnormalities in the lymphoid system rather than from impaired surveillance. The weakened immune response of the patients may even stimulate tumor growth.

In at least one animal model, lack of cell-mediated immunity does not appear to increase the incidence of tumors. Osias Stutman of Memorial Sloan-Kettering Cancer Center, New York City, used a chemical carcinogen to induce cancer in nude mice lacking thymus glands and in nude mice having thymus glands. There were no differences between the two groups either in the length of time before tumors appeared or in tumor incidence. Yet athymic mice do not have active T lymphocytes or cell-mediated immunity.

Not all tumors can stimulate a strong immune response that inhibits tumor growth, according to Prehn. Most of the tumors studied in the laboratory that have this capacity are induced by viruses or chemicals and may be laboratory artifacts. On the other hand, many "spontaneous" tumors have this capability to only a slight degree, if at all. They would not be likely targets for immune surveillance and might elicit only a weak—possibly stimulating—immune response. This argument is double-edged, however. Immune surveillance might be a selective force that favors tumors of low antigenicity by destroying those of higher antigenicity.

Under some conditions, sensitized cells of the lymphoreticular system can stimulate tumor cell division both in vivo and in vitro. In order to cripple the immune responses of mice used for an in vivo study, Prehn first removed their thymus glands and irradiated the animals. Then, he injected them subcutaneously with constant amounts of tumor cells mixed with varying numbers of spleen cells. Large quantities of spleen cells that had been sensitized to the tumor antigens inhibited tumor growth. But small quantities of sensitized cells stimulated tumor growth.

Working in Prehn's laboratory, H. F. Jeejeebhoy injected mice with tumor cells. Lymphocytes taken from the animals before tumors were detectable stimulated division of the corresponding tumor cells in culture. Lymphocytes collected after tumors became detectable inhibited cultured tumor cell division. These results support Prehn's hypothesis that, early in tumorigenesis, a weak immune response is stimulatory while a later, stronger response is inhibitory to tumor growth.

Although Prehn concedes that he is swimming against the tide of opinion about immunosurveillance, he is not alone. Isaiah Fidler of the University of Pennsylvania School of Dental Medicine, Philadelphia, found that small numbers of immune lymphocytes stimulated the growth of cultured tumor cells but a large number of lymphocytes were cytotoxic. The usual in vitro assays, which regularly show cytotoxic effects of lymphocytes, employ high ratios of lymphocytes to tumor cells.

Results from Fidler's laboratory, and from several others, indicate that macrophages may participate in the host's defenses against cancer.

Macrophages from mice that had been immunized against melanoma were cytotoxic to cultured melanoma cells whereas macrophages from normal mice or from mice with growing tumors were not. Fidler could activate macrophages from mice with tumors, however, by incubating them with supernatants from cultures containing both immune lymphocytes and melanoma cells. (Lymphocytes are known to produce factors that activate and attract macrophages.) Fidler thinks macrophage function may be defective in mice with growing tumors. The fact that the defect can be remedied by an in vitro technique suggests another approach to immunotherapy.

In order to act, macrophages must be able to recognize foreign matter. Such recognition depends on the presence of yet another factor—this one called recognition factor. Nicholas DiLuzio and his colleagues at Tulane University, New Orleans, Louisiana, suggest that a failure in recognition mechanisms may contribute to tumor growth and development. They found that carcinoma patients had less recognition factor activity in their serums than did healthy individuals or patients with a number of nonmalignant diseases. Patients with advanced metastatic carcinoma had the lowest levels of all. Recognition factor activity increased following treatment of the carcinoma by surgery or radiation.

DiLuzio thinks that combination of tumor cells with recognition factor may be the first step required for recognition and subsequent attack by macrophages. When he injected leukemic cells into rats, recognition factor activity in serum declined almost 70 percent within 30 minutes, which suggested that the factor had combined with the cells. No decline occurred when normal leukocytes were infused into rats. DiLuzio hypothesizes that failure of recognition mechanisms might permit tumor cells to go undetected by the macrophages and escape destruction.

The Tulane group has isolated and partially characterized recognition factor. It is a protein, an alphaglobulin. DiLuzio, with Peter Mansell, also at Tulane Medical School, initiated clinical trials of the use of recognition factor in cancer therapy. Tumors injected with recognition factor decreased in size. They contained large macrophage populations not seen in uninjected tumors. These observations, although preliminary, support the hypotheses that macrophages and recognition factor are important components of the host's response to tumors.

Not all the pieces of the tumor immunology puzzle have been fitted together. Some are even missing. There are, for example, uncertainties about the specificity of tumor-associated antigens, and about the relation of in vitro assays to in vivo situations. These are more than just technical details, because their interpretation will influence not only the hypotheses formulated about the role of the immune system in oncogenesis but also the strategies devised for immunotherapy. Nevertheless, progress has been made, and investigators are hopeful that the picture is forming.

II
Cancer Biochemistry

6

A Mystery Wrapped in an Enigma

Biochemistry is the darkest recess of cancer research. Less is known about the biochemistry of malignant cells and about differences between malignant and healthy cells, perhaps, than about any other aspect of cancer research. To a great extent, this situation reflects the very small amount of knowledge that is available about the biochemical processes that ensure that the division of healthy cells is halted at an appropriate time. Many biochemists therefore think, according to James D. Watson of the Cold Spring Harbor Laboratory in New York City, that now is not the time to work seriously on the biochemistry of cancer cells: "They argue that, even though cancer cells are the cause of enormous human suffering, nonetheless it does not make sense to put a disproportionate share of our scientific effort into trying to meet an unripe scientific challenge. They compare the current situation with the desire to understand the nature of solar energy at the time of Newton."

Watson himself thinks that such a view may be too pessimistic, but he concedes that there are a great many problems in trying to identify biochemical differences between normal and malignant cells. One of the primary difficulties of this type of analysis, for example, is determining whether an observed change is the primary metabolic disturbance or a secondary response to the primary changes. The problem is compounded in many cases by the difficulties of selecting a good control with which to compare the tumor cell, since it is often unclear what type of normal cell the tumor cell is derived from. The control cells, moreover, often must be isolated normal cells growing in culture. Use of such controls may introduce errors, Watson says, since the normal cells may have undergone many genetic changes during their adaptation to growth in culture.

Even when the control cells are taken from animal tissues, according to Van R. Potter of the McArdle Laboratory for Cancer Research, Madison, Wisconsin, it is difficult to define the "normal" state of the cell. Some enzymes, for example, may be synthesized only during certain stages of the cell cycle and be degraded rapidly thereafter—so they may not be detected if the majority of the cells are at a different stage of the cell cycle. The concentrations of many other enzymes in normal cells vary widely in response to changes in diet, time of day, and the presence of hormones.

Other hazards to meaningful collection of data, Potter says, are found in the conditions for assaying the concentrations of cellular enzymes. Many enzymes—such as phosphofructokinase, carbamylaspartase, and ribotide reductase—are activated or inactivated by minute concentrations of various small, naturally occurring molecules, alone or in combinations. The molecules that exert such allosteric effects frequently are not readily predictable and enzyme assays may be carried out in ignorance of their presence or absence. Another assay hazard, he says, arises because there is often more than one enzyme that catalyzes the reaction on which the assay is based. These may be isoenzymes in the strict sense or they may be more dissimilar enzymes that normally catalyze the same reaction but have different rate and binding constants, as is the case with glucokinase and hexokinase. This problem can be overcome, but only if the presence of the competing enzymes is recognized. Identification of such isoenzymes is, in fact, one of the more fertile areas of research in cancer biochemistry.

Against the backdrop of these problems, a modicum of progress has been achieved. That progress began more than 40 years ago when Otto Warburg and others developed new techniques for measuring metabolic activity within tissues. Examining the limited number of tumors available to him, Warburg discovered that they possessed the unusual trait of producing lactic acid in the presence of oxygen—that is, the tumors metabolized sugar by the normally anaerobic process of glycolysis (fermentation), even though sufficient oxygen should have been available for them to use the aerobic pathways employed in normal cells.

Warburg therefore postulated that malignant cells resulted from a respiratory defect, such as insufficient transport of hydrogen or an inadequate oxidase system. Such a defect has never been documented, however, and many tumors that do not exhibit aerobic glycolysis have subsequently been found. It now appears that aerobic glycolysis occurs in tumors in which the quantity of mitochondria per cell is inadequate in relation to the capacity of the cell to phosphorylate glucose and to carry out glycolysis.

Further studies on the enzymes involved in the oxidative pathways suggested that defects in tumor cells might be explained by any one of a number of defects, alterations, or deletions in the respiratory chain. These observations in the 1940's led the late Jesse P. Greenstein to formulate the theory of convergence. Greenstein postulated that tumor cells tend to converge toward a common pattern of aerobic glycolysis, low concentrations of respiratory enzymes, and a general loss of enzymes not required for the basic existence of the cell—that is, enzymes that carry out the specialized functions of the differentiated cell. The convergence theory is consistent with much current experimental evidence, but there are a great many exceptions to this pattern and the distinction between primary and secondary changes remains unclear.

In the late 1940's, James A. Miller and Elizabeth C. Miller of the McArdle Laboratory demonstrated that certain carcinogenic dyes combine with protein in rat liver and that formation of this carcinogen-protein complex can be correlated with tumor initiation. They coined the term "protein deletion" and postulated that cancer might result from the "alteration or loss of proteins essential for the control of growth but not for life." The protein deletion theory preceded the development of the concepts of repression of genes and feedback control of cellular functions, and the identity of the dye-binding proteins has not yet been determined, but the theory is also consistent with the available experimental evidence.

Extrapolating from these earlier theories, Potter in 1950 suggested that tumor formation might result from an imbalance between the enzymes for anabolism (growth) and those for catabolism (degradation). It is logical, he then argued, that catabolic enzymes are the ultimate regulator of growth; the loss of one or more catabolic enzymes (catabolic deletion) could thus lead to uncontrolled growth. No one has succeeded, however, in identifying a particular catabolic enzyme whose loss is essential to malignant transformation.

Two types of experimental evidence also tend to refute the catabolic deletion theory in its simplest form. First, for every observed deletion there appears to be at least one exception. And second, in regenerating liver, many anabolic enzymes seem to appear only after removal of part of the liver. The new growth could not result simply from loss of a catabolic enzyme because the enzymes necessary for growth did not exist before the partial hepatectomy. Hence, it became apparent that there was a loss of repression of the anabolic enzymes for DNA synthesis and related systems—in general terms, a feedback deletion or modification.

This feedback theory (Figure 15), which has been articulated in the 1960's primarily by Jacques Monod and Francois Jacob of the Pasteur Institute in Paris, is compatible with both the protein deletion theory and the virus theory of cancer. A protein could thus be lost because of a mutation in a structural gene or an altered genome could result from the insertion in the cell of a viral genome with the resultant loss of a specific protein. Alternatively, a target gene could mutate to a form that would be nonreceptive to a repressor protein or a cell membrane could become resistant to passage of a repressor protein.

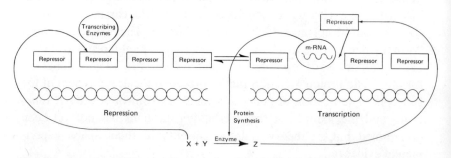

FIGURE 15. One possible simplified mechanism for feedback control of genetic expression. A surplus of the substrate X interacts with the repressor (a histone protein) for the appropriate gene to allow transcription of the gene into messenger RNA (m-RNA). The m-RNA serves as a template for production of the Enzyme that catalyzes the production of Z. Surplus Z then reacts with the initial repressor to shut off the gene.

The altered feedback relations could be caused by a somatic mutation—that is, mutation of a cell other than a germ cell—in which case the change would be irreversible by definition. Or, there could be a feedback alteration without a somatic mutation, in which case the change might be reversible and in some way comparable to differentiation. In any case, it is now a truism that there is some sort of feedback modification present in cancer cells. What remains now is to spell out the details of that mechanism in all their diversity.

7

Biochemistry of Cancer Cells

Focus on the Cell Surface

There is no doubt that cancer cells differ from their normal cell counterparts. What scientists want to identify is the biochemical change (or changes) that produces their altered properties and behavior. The problem is important because identification of such a change may mean that it can be prevented or reversed and malignancy cured. The solution, however, is also elusive, even though it has been the target of considerable scientific enterprise, much of which, during the last 5 years, has been directed at changes in cell membranes following transformation (the conversion of normal cells to cancer cells).

Earlier research frequently centered on the Warburg effect, named after its discoverer, Otto Warburg. Fifty years ago, Warburg observed that tumor cells had a higher rate of glycolysis than did normal cells. Glycolysis is a series of reactions, not requiring oxygen, by which glucose is partially broken down and some of its energy thus recovered for the cell's use. This pathway is an inefficient energy source compared to the aerobic processes that produce most of the energy in normal mammalian cells. Warburg thought that cancer cells originate from normal cells as a result of irreversible damage to their aerobic energy-producing systems and a consequent shift to glycolysis. But the relation between the Warburg effect and transformation is still unclear. Part of the uncertainty, is due to the difficulty—encountered by all investigators studying the differences between normal and cancer cells—in determining whether a particular change, such as the Warburg effect, is a cause or an effect of malignant transformation. Warburg's theory does not account for the aberrant properties of tumor cells. Of these, the capacity to metastasize and the loss of growth control are the most characteristic.

Metastasis is the escape of tumor cells, which appear to be less "sticky" than their normal counterparts, from the tumor mass and their migration to other parts of the body where they may form new tumors. Loss of growth control means that cancer cells continue to divide even under conditions in which normal cells divide only to replace dead cells. This behavior is reflected in vitro by a phenomenon called density-dependent inhibition of growth. In culture, most normal cells stop dividing when they become crowded together; they form a single layer of cells. Transformed cells, on the other hand, continue to divide, piling up layer upon layer of cells (Figure 16).

Because the cell surface membrane is the structure through which cells communicate and interact, both with each other and with their environment, many investigators think that membrane alterations could cause the decreased cellular adhesiveness and loss of growth control seen in tumor cells. Such membrane alterations are thought to be the result of changes in the cell genome, which may be induced by radiation, or by carcinogenic chemicals or viruses, or which may arise spontaneously.

The complexity of mammalian cells is another problem confronting investigators who want to study their biochemistry. Because of it, much remains to be learned about mammalian cell structure and function, especially about the control mechanisms that regulate gene expression and all cell activities. There is, however, a growing realization that membranes, once thought to be relatively inert cell coverings, are dynamic structures that participate in the regulatory mechanisms. The precise role of membranes, in normal cells and especially in transformation, is unclear. Investigators, employing a number of strategies, have detected significant membrane alterations in transformed cells. A unifying concept that explains the membrane's role in transformation has not yet evolved from the different lines of investigation. Instead, there is

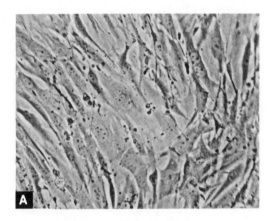

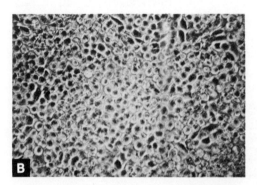

FIGURE 16. Morphological differences between normal and malignant fibroblasts. (A) Normal mouse embryo fibroblasts in culture have a flattened, elongated shape. They grow at a moderate rate, and, as the cells become crowded, their growth rate slows (density-dependent inhibition of growth). (B) Malignant cells, such as these mouse L cells (a highly malignant line of mouse fibroblasts), usually have a more rounded shape. They grow rapidly and are not generally subject to density-dependent inhibition of growth. (C) When the same line of L cells is grown in the presence of a derivative of cyclic AMP, many of the cells revert to a shape and growth pattern more like that of normal cells. [Source: George S. Johnson, Robert M. Friedman, and Ira Pastan, *Proc. Natl. Acad. Sci. U.S.A.* **68**, 425 (1971)]

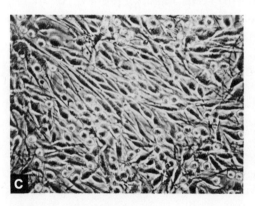

considerable dispute as to what will prove most pertinent to the cancer problem.

Membrane changes in transformed cells can be studied directly by biochemical analysis of important membrane components, such as glycoproteins and glycolipids, or indirectly by using a group of plant proteins called lectins to probe the cell surface. The latter strategy has been employed by a number of investigators, including Garth Nicolson of the Salk Institute, San Diego, California; Max Burger, first at Princeton University, New Jersey, and more recently at the University of Basel, Switzerland; and Leo Sachs, at the Weizmann Institute of Science, Rehovot, Israel. They found that lectins can be used to detect membrane differences between normal and transformed cells. Transformed cells agglutinate in the presence of lectins while the corresponding normal cells, under the same conditions, do not. Agglutination occurs because lectin molecules, which have several binding sites, bind to cell surface receptors—probably the carbohydrate portion of membrane glyco-proteins—on two or more cells and thus cause them to clump.

Nicolson thinks that the greater agglutinability of transformed cells is due to higher mobility of the lectin receptors in cancer cell membranes than in normal cell membranes. With S. J. Singer of the University of California at San Diego, he proposed the fluid mosaic model for the structure of cell membranes. According to this model, the surface membranes of cells are dynamic fluid structures in which membrane components may migrate laterally in the membrane plane (Figure 17).

Using the lectin concanavalin A (Con A) labeled by conjugation to the iron-containing protein ferritin, Nicolson found that the Con A binding sites on the surface of mouse fibroblasts (3T3 cells) transformed by the oncogenic virus SV40 formed clusters more easily than did those on normal 3T3 cells. In some preparations of aggregated transformed cells, he could see clusters of ferritin-labeled Con A at the sites of cell contact.

Nicolson thinks that cluster formation requires migration of the receptors—when transformed cells bind lectins, migration of the recep-tors allows the polyvalent lectins to contact other receptors, form additional linkages, and thus produce clusters of receptors and lectin molecules. This increases local densities of bound lectin molecules so that multiple bridges can form between adjacent cells. Receptors in the

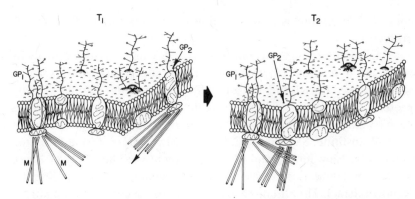

FIGURE 17. Current version of the fluid mosaic model of cell membrane structure. The membrane consists of a lipid bilayer interspersed with glycoproteins (GP) that may penetrate to the inside of the membrane. The carbohydrate portions of the glycoproteins project from the outside. Some of the glycoproteins are free to move laterally while others are restricted in their movements by membrane-associated components (M), possibly microtubules or microfilaments. Under certain conditions, these restricted glycoproteins, GP_2 for example, can be laterally displaced by the membrane-associated contractile components in an energy-dependent process. T_1 and T_2 represent different times. [Source: G. L. Nicolson, *Int. Rev. Cytol.* **39**, 89 (1974)]

membranes of normal cells migrate less readily and do not form clusters well enough for agglutination to occur.

Alterations in the composition of the membrane or in the structure of the lectin receptors following transformation are possible explanations for increased receptor mobility. Nicolson, however, favors the suggestion (made by a number of investigators) that submembrane structures such as microtubules and microfilaments help to regulate the movement of membrane constituents.

Other investigators have found that drugs that disrupt microtubules or microfilaments alter lectin-mediated agglutination of some cells. In order to make contact with submembrane structures, the receptors—glycoproteins in the case of Con A—must penetrate through the double layer of lipids forming the membrane. Many investigators now think that some protein constituents of membranes do extend through the membrane. Thus, there may be connections between membrane glyco-proteins and structures in the cell cytoplasm.

In Sachs' view, agglutination or cell–cell binding requires receptor mobility but not cluster formation. In most experiments, lectin is added to a suspension of cells, which then clump; resolution of the process into discrete steps is not possible. But if the cells could be immobilized to prevent clumping, their response to treatment with Con A and their interaction with other, added cells could be studied in separate operations. Sachs used nylon fibers to which Con A had been covalently linked; cells become immobilized by attaching to the Con A on the fibers. The fiber-bound cells were then treated with Con A and subsequently exposed to the test cells.

As expected, Sachs found that fiber-bound normal lymphocytes bound few normal cells, but fiber-bound lymphoma cells (lymphoma is a type of cancer in which abnormal numbers of lymphocytes are produced by the spleen and lymph nodes) bound large numbers of the tumor cells. An intermediate degree of binding occurred between normal lymphocytes and lymphoma cells.

Treatment of cells with glutaraldehyde fixes the cells and inhibits Con-A-induced agglutination. Glutaraldehyde fixation of both fiber-bound and free test cells prevented cell–cell binding in Sachs' test system. According to Sachs, this indicates that receptor mobility, prevented by the fixation procedure, is required for binding.

If only one cell population (fiber-bound or free) was fixed, however, binding could still occur. Other investigators have found that Con A molecules are held in a diffuse distribution on the surfaces of fixed cells and cannot form clusters. Thus, Sachs concludes that cluster formation is unnecessary for cell–cell binding. He has proposed a model for the mechanism of cell–cell binding induced by Con A. It requires short-range lateral movements of Con A receptors, but not clustering, to allow Con A molecules bound to one cell to find unoccupied receptors on another.

According to Sachs and to M. Inbar and M. Shinitzsky, also at Weizmann Institute, the fluidity of lipids is greater in the membranes of leukemia or lymphoma cells than in normal lymphocytes. Sachs attributes this difference to an increased phospholipid content in leukemia cells and, consequently, a decreased ratio of cholesterol to phospholipids. Inbar and Shinitzsky, on the other hand, found a marked decrease in the cholesterol content of lymphoma cells.

When these investigators artificially increased the cholesterol content of lymphoma cell membranes, the fluidity of the membrane lipids decreased and the cells became less malignant. Animals injected with the treated cells had longer survival times than those injected with untreated cells. Inbar and Shinitzsky suggest that changes in the membrane properties of cells may be involved in conducting specific biochemical signals—such as those regulating cell division—into the cell interior.

The molecular basis of the enhanced lectin agglutinability of transformed cells is as yet unknown, but normal cells can be altered so that they behave more like transformed cells. Max Burger and his colleagues found that mild treatment of normal cells with proteases (enzymes that break down proteins) made them as susceptible as transformed cells to agglutination by lectins. The proteases also stimulated a round of cell division, temporarily releasing the cells from the normal density-dependent inhibition of growth. Burger hypothesizes that derangements in protease activity, especially on membrane components, may be implicated in the development of the characteristics of transformation. The observation by Burger and Hans Schnebli of the University of Basel that protease inhibitors also inhibit the growth of transformed mouse and hamster cells tends to support this hypothesis.

Burger has suggested that transformation produces a conformational rearrangement of the cell surface which exposes hidden receptors and allows them to bind lectin molecules. Transformed cells could then bind more lectin molecules, and, since there would be more opportunities for lectin bridges to form between cells, agglutination would be enhanced. Unlike most other investigators, who have not found such increases, he finds that transformed cells bind three to five times as much lectin as do normal cells. Burger hypothesizes that site exposure results from protease activity.

A variety of changes in membrane structure and function occur in cyclical fashion during the cell cycle. According to Burger, these include an altered response to lectins. He found that normal dividing cells, in contrast to normal nondividing cells, were agglutinated by wheat germ agglutinin. They also bound more lectin molecules than did controls. These and other observations have led Burger to speculate that transformation so alters the cell membrane that it can no longer undergo the normal cyclical changes that terminate cell division—in other words, the cell is effectively trapped in the dividing state.

Increased agglutinability by lectins is not invariably associated with the transformed state. For example, George Poste of Roswell Park Memorial Institute, Buffalo, New York, has shown that infection of normal cells by a number of viruses that are not oncogenic increases the cells' susceptibility to agglutination. The preponderance of evidence, however, does indicate an association between transformation and increased lectin agglutinability, although the mechanism producing enhanced agglutinability is still disputed. Burger favors the hypothesis that increased availability of lectin receptors in transformed cells is responsible, while Nicolson and Sachs, although differing on the necessity for cluster formation, think that increased receptor mobility in such cells is the most important factor.

Analysis of the chemical composition of cells and their membranes is another strategy used by researchers attempting to pin down the differences between normal and malignant cells. Of particular interest are the glycoproteins and glycolipids located in the cell membrane and the enzymes required for their synthesis and breakdown. Glycoproteins and glycolipids consist of a carbohydrate portion plus protein or lipid. The carbohydrates apparently project from the outer membrane surface, where they may be involved in interactions between cells and could be the moieties involved in cell contact and density-dependent inhibition of growth. Lectin receptors are probably glycoproteins.

A number of investigators have found that transformation can alter the composition of membrane glycoproteins and glycolipids. Leonard Warren, Mary Glick, and Clayton Buck of the University of Pennsylvania Medical School, Philadelphia, analyzed glycopeptides removed from cell membrane glycoproteins by the protease trypsin. One fraction of high molecular weight glycopeptides greatly increased in cells transformed spontaneously or by DNA or RNA viruses. The increase appeared to be correlated with transformation, and was not found in cells infected by a nontransforming virus. The increase also occurred in chick embryo fibroblasts infected with a temperature-sensitive mutant of Rous sarcoma virus (RSV) at the permissive temperature but not at the nonpermissive temperature.

Temperature-sensitive mutants such as this RSV mutant (RSV is an oncogenic RNA virus) are proving to be valuable tools for studying transformation. They transform cells at one temperature, the permissive temperature, but not at higher, or nonpermissive, temperatures. Transformation can thus be accomplished at will, simply by adjusting the temperature. The change is reversible, and virus production is maintained at both temperatures. This eliminates the possibility that virus infection rather than transformation produces the effects observed.

According to Warren, Buck, and J. P. Fuhrer, also of the University of Pennsylvania Medical School, the large glycopeptides are formed by addition of sialic acid to precursor glycopeptides. The transfer is catalyzed by an enzyme, a sialyl transferase, whose presence correlates with that of the large glycopeptide fraction.

The function in transformed cells of the membrane glycoproteins from which the glycopeptide fraction is derived is not known. The presence of the glycopeptide fraction depends on cell division, since this fraction is not found in transformed cells that are not dividing. Glick and Buck found a glycopeptide pattern in normal dividing cells similar to that in transformed cells. If the glycopeptides of the two kinds of cells are indeed the same, this would be another resemblance between malignant and dividing cells. Warren says, however, that the large glycopeptides have no measurable affinity for Con A so they are unlikely to be the lectin receptor and thus would not account for the enhanced agglutinability observed by Burger in dividing cells.

Transformation of cells by a chemical carcinogen did not have the same effect on glycopeptides as did viral transformation. Glick, collaborating with Sachs at the Weizmann Institute, observed no differences in the glycopeptide patterns of chemically transformed cells in culture. Cells from tumors that developed in vivo from the transformed cells did have an altered glycopeptide pattern similar to that of virally transformed cultured cells. Moreover, the extent of the change correlated with the cells' tumorigenicity.

Alterations in glycolipid patterns of transformed cells follow a general trend toward simplification; the more complex glycolipids decline in concentration or disappear after transformation. Roscoe Brady and his colleagues at the National Institute of Neurological Disease and Stroke, Bethesda, Maryland, found that certain gangliosides (complex sialic acid–containing glycolipids) disappeared following transformation of mouse cells by DNA viruses. Synthesis of these glycolipids requires sequential addition of sugars and sugar derivatives to the growing molecules. Virally transformed cells lack an enzyme necessary for one of the steps in glycolipid synthesis. Brady did not find these changes in a spontaneously transformed cell line capable of producing tumors in vivo.

Transformation by RNA viruses like RSV also alters the glycolipid pattern of membranes, according to Sen-itiroh Hakomori and his associates at the University of Washington School of Public Health and Community Medicine, Seattle. The concentrations of certain complex glycolipids decreased in transformed chick fibroblasts. The same glycolipids increased when normal cells in culture stopped dividing because of density. Hakomori hypothesizes that these glycolipids form contact-sensitive groups in the cell membrane, which control division. By losing the capacity to synthesize the proper glycolipids at contact, transformed cells escape from density-dependent inhibition of growth. Since some investigators have not found glycolipid changes in transformed cells, Hakomori has suggested that glycoproteins may serve as the contact-sensitive groups in some cell types.

Analysis of cell glycolipids is frequently performed on extracts of whole cells, rather than of membrane preparations. The conclusion that glycolipids are involved in surface phenomena therefore depends on the validity of the assumption that they are located only in the outer membranes. Additional evidence for their involvement has been provided by Hakomori. When he added globoside, a complex glycolipid, to the culture medium of transformed cells it was incorporated into the surface membrane. Moreover, the growth rate of the cells slowed because initiation of DNA synthesis, a prerequisite for mitosis, was delayed.

Another advantage of temperature-sensitive mutants is that they permit identification of very early changes due to transformation—changes that may be causes rather than effects of the altered characteristics of transformed cells. Transformation of cells infected with the mutant begins as soon as they are transferred to the permissive temperature, and they can be studied at short intervals following transfer. Phillips Robbins and Gary Wickus at the Massachusetts Institute of Technology, Cambridge, found an altered protein pattern in the membranes of transformed cells that may be one of the earliest changes of transformation.

According to Robbins and Wickus, a membrane protein with a molecular weight of 45,000 was reduced in amount in chick embryo fibroblasts infected with the temperature-sensitive mutant of RSV and maintained at the permissive temperature but not in the same kind of cells maintained at the nonpermissive temperature. The reduction was associated with transformation rather than with the temperature change; it was found at both temperatures in cells transformed by wild type RSV and at neither temperature in uninfected cells.

The concentration of this protein did not decrease until 3 to 6 hours after transformation was initiated. However, Robbins and Wickus observed a reduction in the concentration of another protein, of as yet uncertain location. This change, also associated with transformation, occurred within 3 hours after transformation was initiated, and may be one of the first effects of transformation.

Other investigators have focused their attention on changes in the enzymes produced by transformed cells. Edward Reich and his colleagues at Rockefeller University, New York City, demonstrated that a number of cultured avian or mammalian cell lines, transformed by either DNA or RNA viruses, produced an enzyme that breaks down fibrin (the protein that forms blood clots) when the incubation media were supplemented with appropriate blood serums. Generation of the fibrinolytic activity required the interaction of two proteins. One is present in normal serums; the other is produced and released into the incubation medium by transformed cells, but not by normal ones.

Reich identified the cell factor as a protease and the serum factor as plasminogen. Plasminogen is the inactive precursor of plasmin, an enzyme that breaks down fibrin. Formation of plasmin normally requires the partial breakdown of plasminogen by a protease; in this case, the protease is secreted by transformed cells.

According to Reich, production of the protease is consistently associated with transformation. When chick embryo fibroblasts were infected with a temperature-sensitive mutant of RSV and cooled to the permissive temperature, appearance of the fibrinolytic activity preceded the morphological evidences of transformation by 4 to 8 hours. When the cells were warmed to the nonpermissive temperature, the fibrinolytic activity declined, which indicated that enzyme production ceased. Alterations of cell morphology resulting from transformation appear to require the action of plasmin. Removal of plasminogen from the incubating serums prevented expression of the alterations.

The role of plasmin in cell transformation is as yet unknown, and Reich prefers not to speculate at this time. However, Burger has implicated proteases in transformation. And Robbins has hypothesized that protease activity could account for the protein loss he saw during transformation. Nicolson considers Reich's contribution significant because it may help explain how cancers metastasize or spread. A protease could enable malignant cells to invade other tissues by breaking down the intracellular matrix or cement that binds cells together. The effect of plasmin on the cell surface membrane will no doubt receive intense scrutiny.

When investigators were looking for a way in which signals regulating cell division might be transmitted from membrane to nucleus or from nucleus to membrane, they turned their attention to that ubiquitous regulator adenosine 3',5'-monophosphate (cyclic AMP) and more recently to guanosine 3',5'-monophosphate (cyclic GMP). Stimulation of cell division is usually associated with low cyclic AMP and high cyclic GMP concentrations or with attainment of the proper ratio of the two nucleotides (*Science*, 12 October 1973). For example, when Burger treated normal cells with proteases and stimulated them to divide, the cyclic AMP concentration declined. Addition of a cyclic AMP derivative during the protease treatment prevented the growth response.

In order to determine what causes the decreases in cyclic AMP after transformation, Ira Pastan and his colleagues at the National Cancer Institute (NCI), Bethesda, Maryland, measured the activity of adenylate cyclase, the enzyme that catalyzes cyclic AMP synthesis, in cells transformed by RSV. They found that its activity declined after transformation. When they infected the cells with temperature-sensitive mutants of RSV and cooled the cells to the permissive temperature, adenylate cyclase activity and the cyclic AMP concentration decreased during transformation. Since adenylate cyclase is a membrane enzyme, Pastan hypothesizes that alterations in membrane glycolipids or glycoproteins caused by transformation affect the enzyme activity and cause a decrease in the cyclic AMP content of the cells.

Whatever the role of cyclic AMP in the mechanism of transformation, there are indications that it can arrest tumor growth in vivo. Pietro Gullino and Yoon Sang Cho-Chung at NCI administered dibutyryl cyclic AMP (an analog of cyclic AMP) to rats with mammary tumors. The tumors stopped growing during the 3 weeks of treatment, and growth resumed when the treatment ceased. Gullino believes that dibutyryl cyclic AMP produced this effect by increasing breakdown of the tumor cells. When the drug was given, the activity of acid ribonuclease, a lysosomal enzyme that breaks down RNA, increased twofold. Gullino had previously shown that regression of certain tumors is accompanied by sharp increases in the activity of six lysosomal enzymes, including acid ribonuclease.

Not all investigators think that cell contact is a significant factor in regulating cell division. Robert Holley of the Salk Institute suggests that growth control of mammalian cells involves interaction among many factors including a number of regulatory agents present in blood serum. He bases his theory partly on his observation that growth of cultured cells depends on the serum concentration of the incubating medium. Normal cells stop dividing at higher densities as the serum concentration increases. Transformed cells, on the other hand, are less dependent on the serum concentration of the medium. They continue to divide even when deprived of serum. Holley has identified four serum factors required for initiating DNA synthesis in normal cells; he is now trying to isolate and characterize them.

In Holley's view, normal cells divide when the intracellular concentration of the necessary nutrients is adequate; they need no additional signals. The availability of these nutrients would be controlled by the serum factors that influence permeability of the cell membrane. Cancer occurs when changes in the membrane release the cells from regulation by the serum factors. Nutrients then enter freely, and cell division becomes continuous. The membrane thus plays a crucial role in oncogenesis, according to Holley's hypothesis, but it is a different role than that proposed by others.

Changes in permeability to the nutrient glucose may be involved in the genesis of the Warburg effect, according to a team of investigators working in Melvin Calvin's laboratory at the University of California at Berkeley. Mina Bissell, James Bassham, and their colleagues found that chick embryo cells transformed by RSV were more permeable to glucose than were their normal counterparts. Since the transformed cells had larger supplies of glucose, some of their metabolic pathways, including glycolysis, proceeded at faster rates than those of normal cells. The Krebs cycle, which utilizes the product of the glycolytic pathway and produces most of the cell's energy, was an exception: It functioned at the same rate in both normal and transformed cells. Although these observations can account for the metabolic changes observed in tumor cells by Warburg, they cannot yet be associated with specific alterations in tumor cell membranes nor do they explain the known properties of tumor cells.

Investigators have found a number of membrane changes associated with transformation—changes in lectin agglutinability, in membrane fluidity, in glycolipid and glycoprotein composition, in proteins, and in enzymes. At present, no one really knows how these observations are related—if they are related. Alterations in membrane composition could affect the fluidity of the membrane or the availability of receptors, or both. So could activity of a protease. Cyclic AMP and GMP may also be involved in the events that regulate cell division. All of this emphasizes the enormous complexity of the mammalian cell and of the problems that must be solved to gain a clearer understanding of the biochemistry of cancer cells.

Most investigators stress that a better understanding of the biochemistry of normal cells, including the mechanisms that regulate gene expression is required. Since their evidence indicates that altered gene expression in transformed cells may be reflected in changes at the cell surface, the relation among genes, membranes, and malignancy provides a promising area for exploration.

8
Fetal Antigens
A Biochemical Assay for Cancer

Perhaps the most crucial deficiency of modern cancer therapy is the difficulty of detecting new tumors at a stage of their development when therapy has a high chance of success. Largely as a result of delayed detection, cancer can now be cured in only one of every three afflicted individuals (where cure is defined as survival for 5 years). This represents an increase of nearly one-third as compared to the cure rate 15 years ago, but some scientists, such as Sidney L. Arje of the American Cancer Society in New York City, suggest that as many as 90 percent of individuals with cancer could be cured with current techniques if tumors could be detected earlier.

A major problem, of course, is that many people receive medical care only irregularly, and there is thus little opportunity for physicians even to attempt detection. By the time these individuals perceive overt symptoms of a tumor, it has generally metastasized (disseminated malignant cells to other sites in the body) and a cure is unlikely. But even when medical attention is available by the time a tumor is large enough to be found by the most commonly used techniques—such as x-rays and palpation of the breasts and prostate— there is a substantial probability of metastasis.

The principal exception to this rule is the Papanicolaou stain (Pap smear), in which cells sloughed from the lining of the uterus are examined for abnormalities indicative of cancer. Increasing use of the Pap smear has lowered the death rate from uterine cancer by 38 percent in 15 years, although only about half of all women in the United States are tested at regular intervals. But the Pap smear represents a unique case in which the sloughed-off cells are readily accessible, and it is unlikely that comparable cytologic assays will be developed for cancers of other internal organs.

It would thus be extremely useful to have biochemical tests that would indicate the presence of a tumor. There are already some enzyme assays that assist in the diagnosis of cancer, points out Oscar Bodansky of the Sloan-Kettering Institute for Cancer Research, New York City. The activity of alkaline phosphatase in the blood, for example, is increased in individuals with skeletal or liver tumors; the activity of acid phosphatase is increased in individuals with prostate tumors. Most assays, though, are less specific for organ site. The activity of glutamate-oxaloacetate aminotransferase, for example, is increased somewhat in nearly every type of cancer, as is the activity of glucose-phosphate isomerase.

These increased activities, which reflect the altered metabolism of tumors, are typically on the order of 10 to 80 percent. Since similar increases are found in many other diseases, these assays are generally not suitable for routine cancer screening. What is required are assays for materials unique to tumors. There has been some progress, particularly with respect to two substances called carcinoembryonic antigen and α-fetoprotein; but there is as yet no biochemical assay for cancer, and there is no prospect for the immediate development and implementation of such an assay. One by-product of research in this area, however, has been a potentially substantive improvement in techniques for assessing the results of cancer therapy.

The search for a biochemical cancer assay has focused primarily on a group of substances known as fetal antigens. (Fetal and other antigens are shown in Figure 18.) These are proteins, glycoproteins, and polysaccharides found primarily in embryonic tissues and fetuses; they are somewhat loosely classified as antigens because of the immune response they provoke in laboratory animals (and, in some cases, in mature animals of the same species). Fetal metabolism is understood only very poorly, but it is clear that fetal tissues contain a large number of enzymes homologous to those in adult tissues. These isoenzymes, or isozymes, perform the same biological functions as those in adult tissues, but have

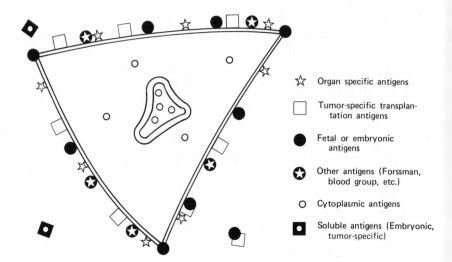

☆   Organ specific antigens

▢   Tumor-specific transplantation antigens

●   Fetal or embryonic
antigens

✪   Other antigens (Forssman,
blood group, etc.)

○   Cytoplasmic antigens

◪   Soluble antigens (Embryonic,
tumor-specific)

FIGURE 18. A schematic representation of antigens which have been identified to exist on rodent tumor cells. [Source: Norman G. Anderson, Oak Ridge National Laboratory]

different amino acid compositions, may have different substrate specificities, are generally subject to different cellular controls, and are immunologically distinct. Fetal cells also contain structural components, particularly glycoproteins, different from those in mature tissues.

It is not clear what advantage the special enzymes provide to embryonic cells, but it seems likely that they are better adapted for the more rapid, sustained growth characteristic of embryos. It is also possible that the fetal structural components play a key role in the embryo's survival in the hostile environment created by its mother's immune system. (Implantation of a fertilized egg in the mother's uterus elicits much the same immune response as does transplantation of an organ, and the fetus survives only by actively interfering with that response.) Once the embryo reaches a certain stage of development, the genes that code for synthesis of the fetal components are in some way deactivated and become part of the cell's large library of dormant genes.

The mammalian genome contains more than 4 billion nucleotide pairs, but only a small fraction of the genes are expressed (transcribed) at any one time. Eric Davidson of the California Institute of Technology, Pasadena, has shown (by molecular hybridization of cellular RNA with

DNA from the genome) that the fraction expressed varies from less than 1 percent in some mature cells to as much as 12 percent in mouse embryos. Since more than 90 percent of the genome must thus normally be kept repressed, there is a great potential for inappropriate expression of genes, particularly if there is interference with the (unknown) chemical regulators of gene expression by carcinogenic chemicals or viruses. Hence it is quite possible that the expression of fetal genes in a mature cell is one cause of cancer.

In this view, espoused by investigators such as Clement L. Markert of Yale University, New Haven, Connecticut, there are no unique properties of cancer cells. Rather, there is only an aggregation of properties not normally found together in mature cells. Two of the three principal characteristics of malignancy—sustained cell division and cell migration—are also characteristic of embryonic cells. The third characteristic is a reversion of structure and metabolic activity to a more primitive or embryonic state. It is thus reasonable, Markert suggests, that cancer simply represents the activity of normal genes functioning in abnormal patterns. This view has only recently begun to be accepted in the United States, where there has been a strong bias toward a viral origin of cancer; it has been much more widely accepted in other countries.

The similarities between malignant and embryonic cells have spurred many investigators to search for common enzymes and structural components which might provide both a way to detect tumors and a means to mount an immunological attack. But this search has been largely a hit-and-miss process, argues Norman G. Anderson, director of the Molecular Anatomy Program at Oak Ridge National Laboratory, Tennessee. What is most urgently needed, he argues, is an organized search for fetal antigens, similar to those for chemical carcinogens and chemotherapeutic agents. Anderson and his associates at Oak Ridge have developed an immunochromatography system to concentrate and isolate the fetal antigens that presumably are present in blood serum, urine, tissue culture supernatants, and tumor extracts. Anderson's system is new and has been little used, but meanwhile the study of fetal antigens has been given some initial momentum by other investigators.

Among the key developments in this research were the discovery of carcinoembryonic antigen (CEA) and α-fetoprotein (AFP). CEA is a glycoprotein that was first isolated from colon tumors in 1965 by Phil

Gold and Samuel O. Freedman of the McGill University School of Medicine, Montreal. AFP, a protein that has long been known to occur in the blood of embryos and infants, was first isolated from liver tumors in 1963 by G. I. Abelov of the N. F. Gameleya Institute for Epidemiology and Microbiology, Moscow. Subsequent investigations have been carried out by many scientists, including Norman Zamcheck of Harvard Medical School, Boston, Massachusetts; Paul Lo Gerfo of the Columbia University College of Physicians and Surgeons, New York City; Thomas A. Waldmann and Richard H. Adamson of the National Cancer Institute, Bethesda, Maryland; Hans Hansen of Hoffman-La Roche Inc., Nutley, New Jersey; E. Douglas Holyoke and T. Ming Chu of the Roswell Park Memorial Institute, Buffalo, New York; and Thomas C. Hall of the University of Southern California, Los Angeles.

The normal functions of CEA and AFP in embryonic tissues are still unknown, but both are relatively abundant. At about the 12th week of gestation, for example, AFP occurs in the blood of a fetus at a concentration of about 1 million nanograms per milliliter. By birth, the concentration has dropped to about 30,000 ng/ml, and in adults it is usually less than 30 ng/ml.

Both CEA and AFP were initially thought to be associated only with fetal tissues and with the specific tumors from which they were first isolated. Many studies have now shown, however, that elevated concentrations of both CEA and AFP are found in the blood of patients with several other types of tumors. More important, these studies have shown that elevated concentrations are not found in all patients with a given type of tumor, and are sometimes found in patients with certain types of nonmalignant disease.

The greatest amount of information is available about CEA, which has been studied in more than 10,000 subjects at some 100 institutions in the United States, Canada, and England. These studies were conducted under the auspices of Hoffman-La Roche as part of its efforts to document the reliability of a radioimmunoassay kit that can be used by practicing physicians to measure CEA concentrations. These studies showed that 97 percent of healthy nonsmoking adults have CEA concentrations in the blood of less than 2.5 ng/ml.

In most patients with tumors, concentrations of CEA were higher than 2.5 ng/ml. Concentrations were elevated in 72 percent of patients

TABLE 2
Typical Carcinoembryonic Antigen (CEA) Concentrations in Patients with Various Diseases
[Source: U.S. Food and Drug Administration]

	Number	Percentage of patients showing CEA at concentrations (ng/ml):			
		0–2.5	2.6–5.0	5.1–10.0	10.0
HEALTHY SUBJECTS					
Nonsmokers	892	97	3	0	0
Former smokers	235	93	5	1	1
Smokers	620	81	15	3	1
CARCINOMAS					
Colorectal	544	28	23	14	35
Pulmonary	181	24	25	25	26
Pancreatic	55	9	31	25	35
Breast	125	53	20	13	14
Other	343	51	28	12	9
NONMALIGNANT DISEASES					
Rectal polyps	90	81	15	3	1
Alcoholic cirrhosis	120	29	44	25	2
Ulcerative colitis	146	69	18	8	5
Emphysema	49	43	37	16	4

with colon and rectal tumors, in 76 percent of patients with lung tumors, and in 91 percent of patients with tumors of the pancreas. But concentrations were also elevated in 19 percent of smokers, 57 percent of patients with emphysema and 71 percent of patients with alcoholic cirrhosis of the liver. Other examples of results from the survey are shown in Table 2. The smaller number of data available for AFP are similar to those for CEA, although the assay is specific for different tumors; most false positive measurements of AFP occur in patients with liver diseases such as hepatitis.

Assays for the two antigens are thus not suitable biochemical tests for cancer, since low concentrations are not proof that a tumor is not there and high concentrations are not proof that it is. The assays are, however, useful as an adjunct to diagnosis by other methods. More important, they are useful in assessing the course of therapy.

Therapy of internal tumors is often a haphazard process since it is generally difficult to ascertain when a tumor has completely disappeared. Chemotherapy, for example, might thus be discontinued too soon, allowing re-emergence of the tumor, or continued for too long, exposing the patient to unnecessary side effects. If a tumor is surgically excised, it is often difficult to know whether all the malignant cells have been removed or whether there have been undiscerned metastases that require further treatment. The antigen assays provide a way to circumvent these problems, and it is for this use that the Hoffman-La Roche assay kit was licensed by the U.S. Food and Drug Administration this year.

Studies by several investigators, especially Zamcheck, Holyoke, Chu, and Waldmann, have shown that when an antigen-producing tumor is surgically removed, the concentration of antigen generally falls to normal levels. Failure of the antigen concentration to decrease or a subsequent increase in the concentration are generally signs that not all of the tumor has been removed and that additional treatment is required. Frequently these recurrent elevated concentrations occur before the new tumor is clinically detectable; they thus offer the potential for follow-up therapy while the new tumor is still small.

In sum, the immediate future looks bright for use of the antigens in assessing therapy, but less bright for their use as a cancer screen. The Hoffman-La Roche studies required more than 4 years to produce a license for limited use of a CEA assay, and it is safe to assume that an antigen for screening would require even more studies. Since there is not now even a candidate antigen for screening, it will apparently be many years before a biochemical assay for cancer will be in use.

III
Cancer Therapy

9
Trends in Cancer Therapy

For decades, cancer therapy has meant surgery, radiation, or both. These therapies will succeed for about one-third of all cancer patients (a total of about 655,000 new cases were diagnosed during 1974), especially when the cancers are detected before they metastasize and seed additional tumors in other parts of the body. But surgery and radiation are limited in that they are suitable only for localized tumors. Certain diffuse cancers, such as the leukemias and lymphomas, are not amenable to these therapies at all. Moreover, metastases, which may be far away from the site of the primary tumor and clinically undetectable, may escape destruction. A single cancer cell left alive can spell a patient's doom.

Some scientists think radiation therapy can be improved by using particulate forms such as high energy neutrons, protons, and alpha particles instead of x-rays or gamma radiation. High-energy particles can deliver a higher dose of radiation to the tumor with less damage to surrounding normal tissue. Even if these types of radiation prove more effective than conventional forms—and they are as yet being investigated only on a relatively small scale—they would still be localized treatments.

Compared to radiation and surgery, chemotherapy, which began to blossom in the 1950's, and immunotherapy, which is just now beginning to be explored in some depth, are newcomers to cancer therapy. Nevertheless, many investigators think that these newcomers, because they are systemic treatments that are at least theoretically capable of reaching—and destroying—cancer cells wherever they lodge in the body, may be the best hope for ultimately achieving cures for the complex of diseases called cancer.

Clinicians visualize a day when systemic therapies will be routinely administered to prevent cancer recurrences in patients whose primary tumors have been surgically removed, even though the patients may appear to be disease-free. At present, immunotherapy is still in the early experimental stages and chemotherapy is used mainly for palliation for patients with advanced disease. The leukemias, lymphomas, and certain other tumors are exceptions. Progress in drug treatment of Hodgkin's disease (a lymphoma) and acute lymphocytic leukemia of children, for example, has spurred research on chemotherapeutic regimens for solid tumors.

Another aspect of the chemical and immunological strategies is their potential use in cancer prevention. This is especially pertinent to cancers that may be caused by viruses (should one ever be unequivocally demonstrated to cause a human cancer). Stimulation of the immune response may bring about destruction of cancer viruses before they cause trouble; alternatively, chemical inhibitors may be found that can prevent the expression of viral genes that turn normal cells into tumor cells. Investigators are also looking for tumor antigens, present on tumor cells but not on normal ones, that could be used to immunize a person against specific cancers, whether or not these have a viral etiology.

Important as these new developments in cancer therapy may be, many experts think that the 5-year survival rate of cancer victims could be increased to 50 percent—or by more than 100,000 people—simply by application of present knowledge. This would involve early detection of the cancers coupled with the best available treatment. The problem is that extending early detection procedures to everyone would severely strain existing health care systems. Thomas H. Ainsworth of the Illinois Masonic Medical Center, Chicago, has estimated that if every physician, including psychiatrists, radiologists, and pathologists, did nothing else, it would still take them $2\frac{1}{2}$ months to give an adequate physical examination to every individual in the United States. The cost would be about 20 billion dollars—about one-third of current annual health expenditures.

This is not to deny the benefits of the campaigns spearheaded by the National Cancer Institute (NCI) and the American Cancer Society to encourage both the medical profession and the lay public to take advantage of techniques for early detection of cancer. For example, NCI attributes the 8-percent decline in the cancer death rate of American women observed over the last 30 years, at least partially, to a sharp reduction in mortality from cancer of the uterine cervix—resulting from early detection of this cancer by means of the Pap smear. The Pap smear is a preparation of cells, normally shed from the cervix that can be examined for atypical cells under the microscope. It even permits detection of abnormal cells that are not yet cancerous but may become so.

With the development and application of more effective techniques for detection and therapy of cancer, an increasing proportion of patients will have their diseases cured or controlled. Many, however, will suffer from residual physical or psychological handicaps that may prevent them from resuming normal lives. For this reason there is growing emphasis on making rehabilitative services available to cancer patients as soon as possible, even while they are still undergoing therapy. Such services would not only reduce the human cost of cancer; they would also reduce the economic cost. The Department of Health, Education, and Welfare estimates that the total cost of cancer during 1973 was $15 billion. Of this $5 billion went for treatment; the remaining $10 billion represents loss of earning power and productivity.

According to John E. Healey, Jr., associate director of the Division of Cancer Control at the University of Miami Comprehensive Cancer Center, Florida, cancer should be considered a chronic disease like diabetes or heart disease. Diabetes and heart disease cannot be cured but they can be controlled, and individuals who have them can lead essentially normal lives. The same should be true of cancer patients.

10
Radiation Therapy
Potential for High Energy Particles

Radiotherapists are among the few cancer clinicians who speak in terms of "cures" rather than the "response rates" or "remission rates" favored by chemotherapists and immunotherapists. This exceptional optimism may be justified. Radiotherapists can, for example, cure 55 to 65 percent of patients with locally inoperable cancer of the prostate and as many as 30 percent of patients with cancer of the urinary bladder, both of which are not susceptible to other types of therapy. In fact, according to Frederick W. George III of the National Cancer Institute (NCI), Bethesda, Maryland, some 60 percent of all cancers are potentially curable with current techniques of irradiation.

But there is a large gap between potential and reality. Presently, only about 33 percent of cancer victims are being cured and that 33 percent includes not only patients treated by irradiation but also those treated with surgery and chemotherapy. Obviously, if George's estimate is correct, current techniques of radiotherapy are not being employed at anywhere near their optimum utility. There appear to be at least four major reasons why this is so. The first is the failure to translate many of the developments in radiotherapy at major cancer centers into the care of the curable patient in the community. A second problem is the inability of physicians to detect the more refractory cancers before they have advanced to the stage of wide dissemination that is beyond control even

100

of the best of cancer centers. The third reason is that large doses of radiation damage healthy tissues in addition to destroying tumors so that, in some cases, at least, the side effects of radiotherapy are potentially as dangerous as the tumor itself. The final reason, intimately related to the other three, is the high cost of research in new techniques of radiotherapy and the limited amount of money that is available for such research.

NCI is attempting to alleviate all of these problems, but perhaps the most promising efforts center on the possibility that the damaging side effects of conventional x-rays and gamma rays can be sharply reduced by the use of high energy particles. Both the physical and radiobiological properties of high energy particles indicate that such particles may be able to alleviate many of the problems of conventional radiotherapy, but extensive clinical trials are needed to ascertain that new and untoward effects do not occur. The potential uses of particle radiation will almost certainly be restricted to localized tumors—a category that, with present methods of detection, generally does not include some of the most common tumors, such as lung and breast tumors. Nonetheless, particle radiation, if its potential advantages turn out to be clinically significant, may be able to help many of the large number of patients who now die from localized cancers despite treatment with conventional radiotherapy.

Practical applications of particle radiation in cancer therapy may be slow in coming. Clinical trials with neutrons have only just begun in this country and the prospects for systematic trials with many other types of particles, while improved, are still modest. Funding for radiotherapy research, including particle radiation, has improved, but is still relatively meager when one considers the large budget of NCI and the apparent potential of radiotherapy. NCI support for investigations of particle radiation has grown from less than $1 million in 1971 to $3.8 million in 1974, a small share of the $30 million budget for radiotherapy and an even smaller share of the $600 million NCI budget. NCI's Radiation Program will, however, receive an additional $4.25 million in 1975 to fund a new radiotherapy development program and much of this funding will be devoted to particle radiation. The impact of the funds for particle radiation has been increased, moreover, by "piggybacking" NCI particle therapy programs on existing accelerators operated by the Department of Defense and the Atomic Energy Commission.

One reason for the relatively slow progress in developing particle radiation, according to NCI, has been the shortage of qualified radiotherapists who are interested and competent in particle radiation. Then too, many research proposals have been rejected in the peer review system for lack of scientific merit—a consequence, it appears, of naiveté in radiobiological matters on the part of the scientists who proposed them. Whatever the reason, some particle accelerators are not being used to their maximum capacity because of insufficient funds and many potential medical applications will be postponed as a result.

The current interest in medical uses for particle radiation contrasts strongly with the attitudes that have prevailed for much of the past 30 years. Early, and what proved to be premature, trials of cancer therapy with high energy neutrons were conducted by Ernest O. Lawrence and his associates at the University of California at Berkeley, in the 1930's. At the time, little was known about the biological effects of radiation and, as a result, the patients were exposed to too large a total dose and a few patients suffered serious delayed side effects. The incident discouraged further work with particle radiation for many years.

More recently, the combination of improvements in conventional radiotherapy techniques—the escalation of x-ray energies from the 200,000 electron volts common in the 1930's to the range of 4 to 35 million electron volts in use now, and the use of gamma rays—and the sharply limited availability of experimental time at major accelerators because of the higher priority that was given to physics experiments provided little incentive for radiobiological investigations with heavy particles. Nevertheless, considerable work was done with obsolete machines at a few laboratories, notably at Berkeley and at Harvard, Cambridge, Massachusetts. In the last 5 years, however, physics research funds have grown much more scarce; quite a few accelerators have become available, and this phenomenon has combined with the lure of technological breakthroughs in radiotherapy to create something of a rush for physicists to get into cancer research. Neutrons, protons, alpha particles (helium ions), heavy ions such as nitrogren or neon, and the pi minus meson, or pion, are among the particles being considered for radiotherapy.

Compared to 30 years ago, considerably more is known now about the effects of radiation on tissue. Two factors in particular seem to be important to the prospects of particle radiation: (i) the dose delivered to the tumor in comparison to that inflicted on healthy tissue; and (ii) the biological effectiveness of the radiation in the tissue.

X-rays and gamma rays interact with electrons as they travel through tissue so that their energy is attenuated exponentially. Except for a small buildup just beneath the tissue surface, the energy transmitted to the tissue decreases with depth. A deep-seated tumor thus receives a smaller dose than does the healthy tissue above it. The tissue behind the tumor also receives a substantial, although smaller dose.

Heavy charged particles also lose energy in tissue by scattering electrons, but, in contrast to x-rays and gamma rays, their energy loss occurs at a rate proportional to the square of their nuclear charge and inversely proportional to their energy (at velocities much less than the speed of light). A nearly constant amount of radiation, therefore, is deposited along most of the path of the particle. As the particle comes to a stop, however, the amount of radiation deposited rises sharply to a maximum (Figure 19) known as the Bragg peak. If the initial energy of a beam of charged particles is adjusted so that the Bragg peak occurs in the tumor, the intervening normal tissue above the tumor receives less radiation than does the tumor. Tissues behind the tumor receive almost no radiation since most of the particles stop in the tumor.

Hence, charged particles, because they allow the radiation to be concentrated in the tumor, appear to be an improvement over conventional radiotherapy. That this improvement in dose localization is clinically significant has not been fully demonstrated and some radiotherapists remain skeptical. But the successful use of high energy x-rays and gamma rays, both of which have better dose localization than do low energy x-rays, suggests that the concept is sound.

The amount of radiation delivered to the tumor is not the only consideration, however, because the biological response of cells to radiation varies with the condition of the cell and the type of radiation. Many tumors, for example, appear to be undifferentiated tissue that has an inadequate blood supply and hence may contain a small proportion of cells that have a lower than normal concentration of oxygen. With conventional radiation, the dose required to kill such oxygen-poor cells is as much as three times that which will destroy normal, oxygenated cells—an effect that is believed by many radiotherapists to be due to the

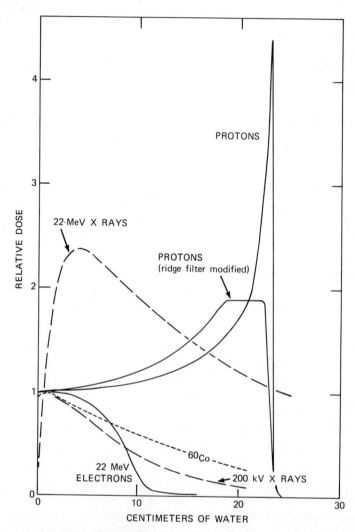

FIGURE 19. Energy transfer as a function of depth for several types of radiation. The curves for protons are similar to those for other heavy ions. [Source: M. R. Raju, Lawrence Berkeley Laboratory]

high reactivity (within normal cells) of the free radicals created when unbound oxygen is ionized by the radiation. The radiosensitivity of cells also appears to vary with cell cycle, although less is known about why this should be so. Both these effects may make tumors less susceptible to radiation than is normal tissue. The magnitude of both these effects, however, seems to be less with particle radiation than with conventional radiation.

The greater effectiveness of particle radiation in destroying tumor cells—and its potentially lesser dependence on the cell's oxygen content or cycle—is apparently due to the higher density of ionization, compared to x-rays, that the particles produce in tissue. The higher the ionization density, or the amount of energy transferred to the tissue per unit of path of a particle (linear energy transfer, or LET), the greater the tissue damage. The greater effectiveness of high LET radiation for some types of tumor systems has been demonstrated in animal studies. But whether anoxic tissue is a significant factor in human tumors and whether the oxygen effect is a limiting factor in radiation therapy remain to be clinically proved.

One indication that high LET radiation may indeed be effective in human tumors comes from clinical trials of fast neutrons at the Hammersmith Hospital in London. After several years of careful and detailed radiobiological studies, in 1969 Mary Catterall and her associates at the hospital began investigating the effects of neutrons on human tumors. Preliminary trials with a neutron beam (obtained by bombarding a beryllium target with high energy deuterons) showed that the responses of patients treated with neutrons did not differ in any observable way from those of patients treated with x-rays. The reaction of the patients' skin to a total dose of about 1440 rads of neutron radiation, however, was judged to be about the same as that produced by 4100 rads of high-voltage x-rays.

Neutrons are like electrons in that their energy is attenuated exponentially with depth in tissue. The destruction of tumor cells by neutrons, however, appears to be only about half as sensitive to the oxygen content of the cells as that caused by x-rays. Clinical trials with more than 300 patients at Hammersmith indicate that this oxygen effect may be very significant clinically; after irradiation, there appear to be remarkably few recurrences of tumors in neutron-treated tissue among the surviving-patients. One U.S. radiotherapist who is familiar with the work has described it as "startling, if the preliminary indications hold up."

The advantage of neutrons over conventional radiation may, however, be dependent on the type of tumor and its growth rate. Less extensive trials by G. W. Barendson and his associates at The Radiobiological Institute in Rijswijk, the Netherlands, for example, suggest that neutrons may be no more effective than cobalt-60 radiation in treating certain lung tumors. More information about the potential for neutron irradiation will be obtained only from much more extensive clinical trials, which have begun only within the last year.

In the United States, such trials are being conducted at three locations: the University of Washington, Seattle, under the direction of Robert S. Parker; M. D. Anderson Hospital and Tumor Institute, Houston, Texas, under the direction of Gilbert Fletcher and David Hussey; and a cooperative program at the Naval Research Laboratory, Washington, D.C., under the direction of Charles C. Rogers of George Washington University, Washington, D.C. These programs have already treated a total of more than 600 cancer patients, but little assessment of their results is possible until adequate data about the survival of the patients is accumulated, a process that may take 5 years or longer.

Even then, the results may not be definitive: Most of the first cancer victims to be treated with neutron radiation are terminal patients for whom all other types of therapy are ineffective. A clear improvement in these patients will be firm evidence that neutron radiation therapy is effective, but the absence of improvement might mean only that the therapy is just effective against less-advanced tumors, as is the case with chemotherapy. The trials will, however, indicate whether there are any serious side effects to the therapy. In anticipation that the trials will be successful, meanwhile, other investigators, such as James T. Brennan of the University of Pennsylvania, Philadelphia, are working on the development of more economical neutron sources, suitable for use in hospitals, to replace the expensive cyclotrons.

Unlike the case with neutrons, the damage caused to tumors by protons has about the same sensitivity to cell oxygen content as that caused by conventional radiation. Because of the Bragg peak effect, however, protons are superior to neutrons in localizing the dose within the tumor. The proton beam can be focused so sharply, in fact, that a major limitation in making use of protons is the lack of a sufficiently accurate means of locating tumors within the body—techniques for which there is little need with the broad beams used in conventional radiotherapy. Nonetheless, therapeutic work with protons has been conducted at Berkeley, Harvard, and the University Hospital in Uppsala, Sweden, for more than a decade, primarily for the treatment of conditions (such as acromegaly, Cushing's disease, and Nelson's disease) that require destruction of the pituitary gland.

There have been no full-scale clinical trials with protons against tumors, but there have been some preliminary experiments. Herman D. Suit of Harvard, for example, has used protons for the treatment of retinoblastoma (a tumor of the eye) and certain types of sarcoma that had previously been thought to be resistant to radiation. There has been a low incidence of serious side effects associated with proton radiation. One further advantage of protons is their low cost: The Harvard cyclotron has been supported since 1967 largely by patient fees for pituitary irradiation.

Some of the advantages of both protons and neutrons can apparently be obtained by using alpha particles, ions containing two protons and two neutrons. The energy transfer of alpha particles is concentrated in a pronounced Bragg peak, as with protons, and the oxygen dependence within the peak is nearly as low as that of neutrons. The Bragg peaks of alpha particles are extremely narrow, however, and a large tumor cannot be completely irradiated unless the range of the beam is varied or the width of the peak is broadened by inserting a variable absorber in the path of the beam.

It had been thought that broadening the Bragg peak might destroy the low oxygen dependence of alpha particles. But M. R. Raju of the Lawrence Berkeley Laboratory has shown that, with cultured cells, at least, that is not the case. Systematic clinical trials with alpha particles have not yet begun, although alpha particles produced by the 184-inch cyclotron at Berkeley have been used since 1956 for pituitary irradiation. Several other accelerators that can produce alpha particles of sufficiently high energy for cancer therapy are now available.

Neutron, proton, and alpha particle accelerators that would be suitable for clinical studies are already available and substantial information about the radiobiological behavior of these particles has already been obtained. Much less is known about heavy ions and pions and their presumed relative advantages are unproved in practice. Nonetheless, many radiotherapists are firmly convinced that such particles have significant potential for application against tumors.

Heavy ions with energies suitable for radiobiological studies have become available only recently. In 1971, Cornelius A. Tobias of Berkeley and his associates produced high energy beams of nitrogen nuclei. Subsequently, they have produced similar beams of carbon, oxygen, and neon ions. These heavy ions are of interest because they have exceptionally intense Bragg peaks—an indication of potentially high biological efficacy. What is not known, however, is the extent to which that efficacy will be decreased when the Bragg peak is broadened to widths comparable to those of real tumors. And very little is known about the physics of heavy ions—including what secondary particles are produced in tissue. The Berkeley accelerator has recently been modified to improve its capability for acceleration of heavy ions, however, and some of the necessary information should be forthcoming.

Also completed recently are three new facilities for the production of pi minus mesons, or pions—short-lived, (mean lifetime, 2.54×10^{-8} seconds), negatively charged particles with a mass 273 times that of an electron (or 15 percent that of a proton). These are the Atomic Energy Commission's Los Alamos Meson Physics Facility in New Mexico and similar installations at the Tri-University Meson Facility in Vancouver, British Columbia, and the Swiss Institute for Nuclear Research in Zurich, Switzerland. Stanford University has also completed a superconducting electron accelerator that could be used to produce pions. The Los Alamos facility includes a special beam channel for therapeutic work built with support from NCI.

These expensive installations are required because of the low efficiency of pion production. Pions are obtained by bombarding a beryllium target with high energy protons (Figure 20), but only 1 pion is obtained for every 10^5 to 10^6 protons accelerated. A very large flux of protons is thus needed for formation of a therapeutically effective beam.

Pions with an appropriate initial energy pass through the tissue surrounding a tumor with exceptionally low damage. As they slow down in the tumor, however, they are captured by carbon, nitrogen, and oxygen

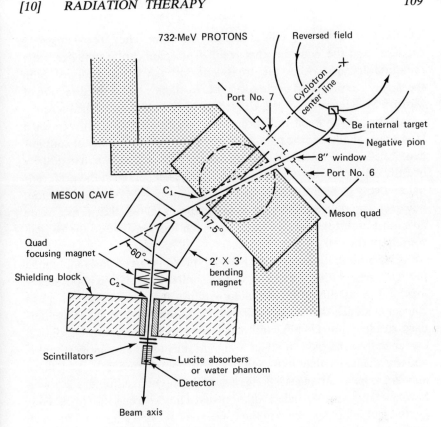

FIGURE 20. A typical experimental setup for generating pions. [Source: M. R. Raju, Lawrence Berkeley Laboratory]

atoms. The capture process produces x-irradiation and a localized burst of secondary particles. Each pion capture produces, on the average, one proton or deuteron, one alpha particle, one particle with an atomic number of three or more, and three neutrons. The radiation dose contributed locally by the neutrons is relatively small. The protons contribute substantially more radiation but, according to Raju, the greatest biological effect is produced by the alpha particles, which have an average range of about 8 micrometers.

The net effect is that pions, like heavy ions, deposit a highly localized radiation dose that is theoretically very effective biologically, although by a mechanism different from that which causes the Bragg peak of a heavy ion. Pions have two major disadvantages, however. They are expensive to produce, and the neutrons that result from pion capture may create a radiation hazard within the treatment room. Clinical trials of pion therapy are expected to begin soon at Los Alamos under the direction of Morton M. Kligerman of the University of New Mexico, Albequerque.

With conventional radiation, then, healthy tissue often receives a larger dose than does the tumor and, to the extent that the tumor contains anoxic cells, it takes more radiation to destroy tumor cells than to destroy healthy cells. Conventional radiotherapy thus depends on the preferential recovery of healthy tissue for its success. Charged particle radiation, however, can deliver higher doses to the tumor than to the normal tissue around it and, for some particles, is much less sensitive to the oxygen content of the cell.

The radiobiological properties of protons, neutrons, and alpha particles are relatively well known and similar information about heavy ions and pions should be available within a few years. There is much clinical evidence that dose localization is important and, if the preliminary results from Hammersmith are confirmed, there will be clinical evidence that the oxygen effect is significant in human tumors (there is already evidence that it is significant in animal tumors). And there appears to be a consensus among radiobiologists and radiotherapists who have worked with particle radiation that clinical trials should be conducted with all types. Among the cancers most often suggested for such trials are tumors of the oral cavity, the bladder, the cervix, and the pancreas.

Even ardent supporters of particle radiotherapy agree, however, that it would be a mistake to divert too much money from basic cancer research to the sophisticated technologies required for studying the effects of particle radiation. Miracles are not likely, they caution, but the evidence so far suggests that particle radiation therapy is well worth trying.

11
Chemotherapy
Now a Promising Weapon

Chemicals have made a substantial contribution to cancer therapy during the past 20 years. In 1954, one of every four patients afflicted with cancer could expect to have his survival extended for 5 years or more by effective therapy. Today, the proportion of patients so "cured" has risen to one in three and is still climbing, even if slowly. A substantial fraction of this nearly 30 percent increase in the cure rate, which amounts to 55,000 additional lives saved each year, can be attributed to advances in cancer chemotherapy.

Surgery and radiation are, of course, still the primary forms of cancer therapy. Surgery, the weapon most widely used for a first attack on tumors, is remarkably successful in certain types of malignancies. It is the primary factor responsible for extending survival to 5 years in more than 85 percent of patients with skin cancer, in about 60 percent of women with breast cancer, in about 40 percent of patients with cancer of the colon, and in about 70 percent of women with cancer of the uterus.

Radiation is the second most important weapon in the therapist's arsenal. It is particularly useful for treating internal solid tumors if they are detected at an early stage of development. When such tumors are caught early, radiotherapy is responsible for extending survival to 5 years in at least 90 percent of men with one type (seminoma) of cancer of the testis, in at least 80 percent of children with retinoblastoma (a cancer of

TABLE 3
The Susceptibility of Certain Tumors to Chemotherapeutic Agents
[Source: Irwin H. Krakoff, Memorial Hospital for Cancer and Allied Diseases, New York City]

Type of cancer	Useful drugs	Results
PROLONGED SURVIVAL OR CURE		
Gestational troplastic tumors	Methotrexate, Dactinomycin, Vinblastine	70% cured
Burkitt's tumor	Cyclophosphamide (many others)	50% cured
Testicular tumors	Dactinomycin,* Methotrexate,* Chlorambucil*	30–40% respond, 2-3% cured
Wilms' tumor	Dactinomycin with surgery and radiotherapy	30–40% cured
Neuroblastoma	Cylophosphamide with surgery and/or radiotherapy	5% cured
Acute lymphoblastic leukemia	Daunorubicin,* Prednisone,* Vincristine,* 6-Mercapto-purine,* Methotrexate,* BCNU*	90% remission, 70% survive beyond 5 years
Hodgkin's disease Stage IIIB & IV	HN2,* Vincristine,* Prednisone,* Procarbazine,* Bleomycin	70% respond, 40% survive beyond 5 years
PALLIATION AND PROLONGATION OF LIFE		
Prostate carcinoma	Estrogens, castration	70% respond with some prolongation of life
Breast carcinoma	Androgens, estrogens, alkyl-ating agents,* 5-Fluorour-acil,* Vincristine,* Prednisone,* Methotrexate*	20–40% respond with probable prolongation of life
Chronic lymphocytic leukemia	Prednisone, alkylating agents	50% respond with probable prolongation of life
Lymphosarcoma	Prednisone, alkylating agents	50% respond with probable prolongation of life
Acute myeloblastic leukemia	Arabinosylcytosine and Thioguanine	65% remission with prolongation of life
PALLIATION WITH UNCERTAIN PROLONGATION OF LIFE		
Chronic granulocytic leukemia	Alkylating agents, 6-Mercaptopurine	90% respond with good control during most of course
Multiple myeloma	Alkylating agents	36% respond objectively, 50% have subjective relief of symptoms
Ovary	Alkylating agents	30–40% respond
Endometrium	Progestins	25% respond, chiefly pulmonary metastases

*May be used in combination.

TABLE 3 continued

Type of cancer	Useful drugs	Results
UNCERTAIN PALLIATION		
Lung	Alkylating agents	30–40% respond briefly
Head and neck	Alkylating agents, Methotrexate	20–30% respond briefly
Large bowel	5-Fluorouracil	10–20% respond
Stomach	5-Fluorouracil	10% respond
Pancreas	5-Fluorouracil	<10% respond
Liver	5-Fluorouracil	<10% respond
Uterine cervix	Alkylating agents	<10% respond
Melanoma	Alkylating agents, Vinblastine	<5% respond
Adrenal cortex	o,p'-DDD	Relief of Cushingoid syndrome
Soft tissue and osteogenic sarcoma	Adriamycin, Methotrexate	20% respond
LOCAL CHEMOTHERAPY TECHNIQUE		
Intracavarity injection for recurrent effusion	Alkylating agents, 5-Fluorouracil, Quinacrine	50% of effusions controlled
Intrathecal injection for meningeal leukemia	Methotrexate, Arabinosylcytosine	80% improved—2 months
Extracorporeal perfusion for cancer of extremities	Alkylating agents	Irregular and uncertain
Continuous infusion for cancer of head and neck, liver, and pelvis	Methotrexate-Leucoverin, 5-Fluorouracil	Irregular and uncertain

the eye), in about 75 percent of patients with Hodgkin's disease (a cancer of the lymph system), and in about 50 percent of patients with cancer of the nasopharynx.

Both surgery and radiotherapy, however, have been near the limits of their utility for many years, especially since they are generally useful only against localized tumors. There is some possibility that major improvements in radiotherapy may result from improvements in focusing the radiation dose on the tumor and from the exploitation of alternative forms of radiation such as fast neutrons and negative pi mesons. Nonetheless, the therapeutic efficacies of surgery and radiation are little different from what they were 20 years ago; the only substantive difference is that they are now employed in the treatment of a larger number of patients than earlier.

The situation is substantially different in chemotherapy. In 1954, shortly before the direction of cancer chemotherapy was consolidated in what is now the Division of Cancer Treatment of the National Cancer Institute (NCI), Bethesda, Maryland, there were perhaps a half-dozen anticancer drugs in clinical use, and there were no types of cancer in which drugs could produce substantive improvements in large numbers of patients. Today, there are approximately 40 active drugs that are being used to treat cancer, 10 or so for which clinical testing has recently begun, and another 30 that are in earlier stages of testing. There are also at least 10 types of cancer (out of more than 100) in which it appears that a significant proportion of patients can have their survival extended to at least 5 years with drugs, and the median period of survival is increasing in a number of others (Table 3). Progress in the discipline has been relatively slow—some physicians would say agonizingly slow—and there are some crucial stumbling blocks that must be overcome, but the future has never looked brighter or more full of hope.

Despite these successes, cancer chemotherapists have a lingering poor reputation among large segments of the lay public. The many apparent failures of chemotherapeutic agents during the 1950's were a bitter disappointment to a public that had rapidly grown accustomed to "miracle" cures of bacterial diseases by the recently discovered antibiotics. This bitterness was compounded by the severe side effects associated with many of the most potent anticancer agents, side effects that were frequently given more weight in the public consciousness than the definite palliative effects.

To a great extent, the early failures and the accompanying disappointment resulted from an experimental approach dictated by ethical considerations. The untried anticancer agents could be used only as a last resort in patients for whom all other types of therapy had failed. In most such cases, the patient had already been subjected to surgery, radiotherapy, or both, and the tumor burden was so overwhelming that it was remarkable that the drugs could have any effect at all. All too frequently, friends and relatives of the patients viewed the prolongation of suffering and the side effects of the drugs as a cruel hoax, and that viewpoint has left a residuum of bitterness and skepticism toward chemotherapists. But the investigations of those early years laid a strong foundation for the successes that were to come more recently.

Significantly, many of the earliest successes were obtained with cancers for which the prognosis was most hopeless. These included particularly the leukemias and lymphomas, hemopoietic cancers (cancers of the blood-forming organs) in which malignant white blood cells produced by the bone marrow and the lymph glands, respectively, are disseminated throughout the body. Since these malignancies are generally not susceptible to surgery or radiotherapy and were always fatal, chemotherapists were able to initiate treatment as soon as the tumors were diagnosed and, therefore, while the tumor burden was relatively small.

Malignant cells in the hemopoietic cancers also have a growth rate much higher than that of most normal cells (and most tumor cells), and this difference provided the key point of attack. Chemotherapists were thus able not only to treat these malignancies successfully, but also to establish several principles of chemotherapy that have only recently begun to be applied to other types of tumors.

Perhaps the most important of these principles is that chemotherapy has its greatest chance of success when it is applied aggressively against small tumors that have only recently become established; it is much less effective against tumors that are older and larger. This is true whether chemotherapy is the only form of treatment or whether it is used in combination with other techniques. Almost equally important, investigators have shown that appropriate combinations of drugs are, if not synergistic, at least significantly more effective than single agents.

It is extremely difficult to assign credit fairly for the development of these concepts. In the first place, there is an exceptionally large number of people working in chemotherapy. Second, the concepts that have proved most important have evolved slowly from the independent work of many investigators. And finally, since many of the tumors that are most susceptible to chemotherapy are among the rarer forms of cancer, clinical trials of promising drugs and treatment regimens frequently require the cooperation of clinicians at many institutions.

Nevertheless, it is possible to select a few names of individuals who have played crucial roles in establishing the principles of combination chemotherapy, early chemotherapy, and chemotherapy as an adjuvant to other types of treatment. These would include: Emil Frei III of the Children's Cancer Research Foundation, Boston, Massachusetts; Emil J.

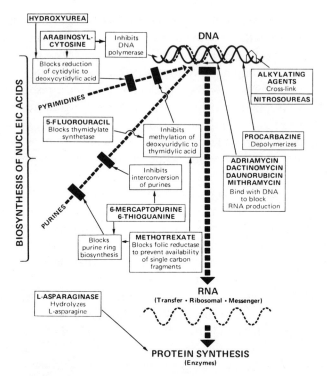

FIGURE. 21. The mechanism of action of several antitumor agents that interfere with the replication of cells. [Source: Irwin H. Krakoff, Memorial Hospital for Cancer and Allied Diseases, New York City]

Freireich of the M. D. Anderson Hospital and Tumor Institute, Houston, Texas; James F. Holland of the Mt. Sinai School of Medicine, New York City; Joseph H. Burchenal of Memorial Sloan-Kettering Cancer Center, New York City; Howard E. Skipper and Frank Schabel, Jr., of the Southern Research Institute, Birmingham, Alabama; and C. Gordon Zubrod, Abraham Goldin, Paul P. Carbone, and Vincent T. DeVita, Jr., of NCI.

There are a number of substantive biological differences between old and young tumors that explain why older tumors are more refractory to chemotherapy; many of these differences have been elucidated by Skipper and Schabel. Perhaps the most important difference is that most of the cells in a very young tumor are continually passing through the mitotic cycle for replication—that is, the young tumor has a large fraction of actively growing cells. Since most current antitumor drugs act by interfering with this cycle (Figures 21 and 22), this large growth fraction makes the cells highly susceptible to the killing effects of antitumor drugs.

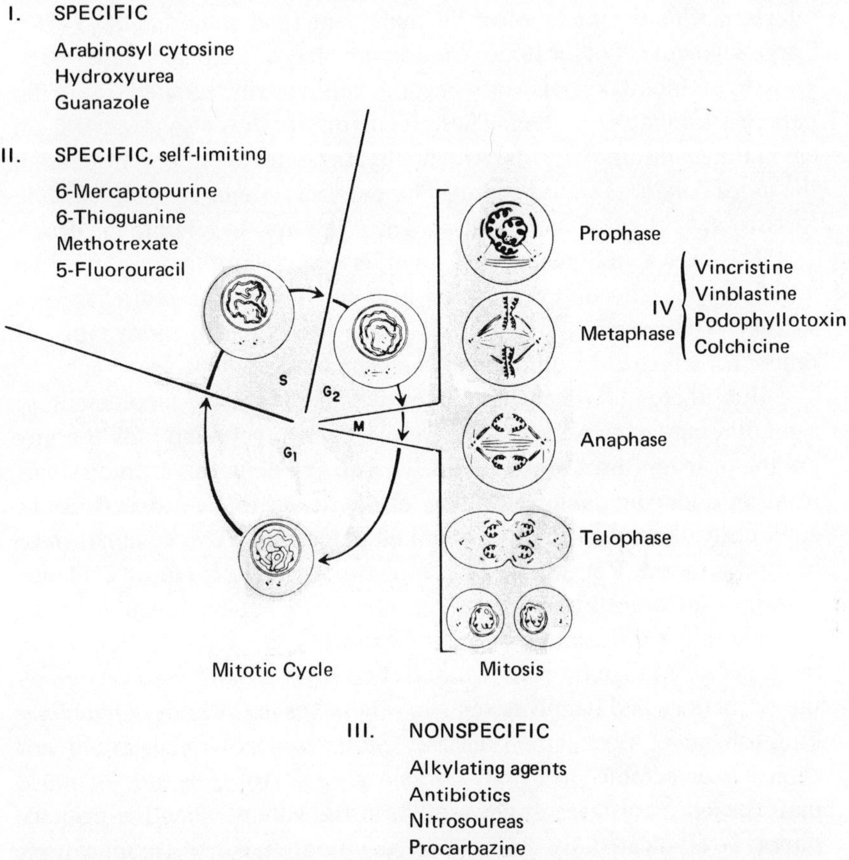

I. SPECIFIC

    Arabinosyl cytosine
    Hydroxyurea
    Guanazole

II. SPECIFIC, self-limiting

    6-Mercaptopurine
    6-Thioguanine
    Methotrexate
    5-Fluorouracil

Prophase

$$IV$$ Metaphase
    Vincristine
    Vinblastine
    Podophyllotoxin
    Colchicine

S G_2 M G_1

Anaphase

Telophase

Mitotic Cycle   Mitosis

III. NONSPECIFIC

    Alkylating agents
    Antibiotics
    Nitrosoureas
    Procarbazine

FIGURE 22. Chemotherapeutic agents interfere at different phases of the mitotic cycle. (I) Drugs whose sole or principal mechanism of action is inhibition of DNA synthesis interfere in the S-phase, where DNA synthesis occurs. (II) Some inhibitors of DNA synthesis also inhibit RNA and protein synthesis. These last effects slow the cell cycle and prevent cells from entering the highly sensitive S-phase. (III) Some chemotherapeutic agents exert a direct effect on DNA and their activities are not enhanced by administration during S-phase. (IV) Some agents, all plant alkaloids, have the ability to arrest mitosis in metaphase. [Source: Irwin H. Krakoff, Memorial Hospital for Cancer and Allied Diseases, New York City]

In older tumors, in contrast, there is a much smaller growth fraction and the tumor is much less susceptible to chemotherapy.

There are also proportionately many more dead cells in a larger tumor; these cells release metabolites that may fuel adjacent viable cells, and inhibit the action of antimetabolites, a class of antitumor agents that interfere with the metabolism of malignant (and some healthy) cells. Large segments of older tumors, moreover, may occasionally outstrip the growth of blood vessels and become temporarily isolated from the patient's circulatory system. These segments are thus also isolated from circulating antitumor agents. And finally, the older the tumor, in general, the more debilitated the patient is; his defense systems are thus less able to assist in fighting off the tumor, and he is less able to tolerate the drug.

The inescapable conclusion, then, is that chemotherapy should be initiated while the tumor is young in order to have the best chance of success. This conclusion has been readily accepted in those types of cancer for which chemotherapy is the primary treatment.

But there has been great reluctance to use supplementary chemotherapy in those types of cancer where surgery and radiotherapy are the primary forms of treatment. To a large extent, this attitude stems from an understandable reluctance of physicians to give toxic drugs to apparently healthy patients in whom all detectable traces of tumor have been eradicated. Yet in many types of cancer, there is strong evidence that these apparently healthy patients are not free of malignant disease.

The most devastating aspect of cancer is the ability of tumors to metastasize: Malignant cells are detached from a tumor and carried by the circulatory and lymph systems to other sites in the body, where they establish small pockets of disease. Since tumors are generally not clinically detectable until they contain at least 10^9 cells, one or more undiscerned metastases might remain in the patient when the primary tumor is eradicated by surgery or radiation. It is the complications associated with the subsequent growth of these metastases that are responsible for the majority of cancer deaths. A growing number of clinicians, consequently, have begun arguing that these metastases should be attacked aggressively with chemotherapy before they are clinically detectable and while they are still most susceptible to drug treatment.

This type of adjuvant chemotherapy has been attempted in the past—particularly in breast cancer patients in the late 1950's—with generally disappointing results. Some scientists, such as Memorial Sloan-Kettering's Burchenal, argue that those failures were due mainly to the use of relatively inactive drugs given for too short a time and in inadequate doses. The current knowledge of treatment regimens, he insists, gives adjuvant chemotherapy a much greater potential for success.

A major problem, however, is identifying those high-risk patients for whom the potential benefits of chemotherapy outweigh the risks. The need for such identification is one explanation for the intense interest in the development of sensitive assays for the detection of biochemical markers or of fetal and tumor antigens from tumors that would otherwise be undiscernible. Such assays would also be extremely useful in monitoring the course of chemotherapy. Their development, argues NCI's Zubrod, director of the institute's Division of Cancer Treatment, would do more to speed the chemical control of cancer than any other single technique. In the interim, however, clinicians are forced to rely on past experiences to predict which patients are the best candidates for adjuvant chemotherapy. Typically, these have been patients in whom a fatal recurrence was a foregone conclusion. Good examples of the recent successes of aggressive chemotherapy against such malignancies are provided by results with several childhood tumors, including Wilms' tumor, embryonal rhabdomyosarcoma, and osteogenic sarcoma.

Wilms' tumor is a lethal cancer of the kidney of children. Treatment with either surgery or radiation has produced cure rates (2-year survival) no higher than 23 percent; a combination of the two increases the rate to 40 percent. But the late Sidney Farber and his associates at the Children's Cancer Research Foundation have shown that the cure rate can be increased to more than 80 percent if surgery and radiotherapy are followed by treatment with the antitumor antibiotic actinomycin D. Even if lung metastases are present when the tumor is discovered, they found that radiotherapy and actinomycin D provide nearly 50 percent long-term (5 years) survival.

Embryonal rhabdomyosarcoma, a muscle tumor that generally appears soon after birth, exhibits much the same responsiveness to surgery and radiation as does Wilms' tumor, but is less sensitive to chemotherapy. Nonetheless, Charles B. Pratt III of St. Jude Children's Research Hospital in Memphis, Tennessee, Sarah S. Donaldson and J. R.

Wilbur of Stanford University School of Medicine in Palo Alto, California, and Fersteh Ghavimi of Memorial Sloan-Kettering have shown that surgical removal of the bulk of the tumor, radiation therapy to all known areas of disease, and as much as 2 years of chemotherapy with a combination of vincristine, actinomycin D, and cyclophosphamide appears to produce long-term, disease-free survival. Donaldson and Wilbur report that 14 of 19 patients have no evidence of disease 3 to 10 years after the start of therapy. Ghavimi has obtained similar results in 21 of 25 patients observed for as long as 3 years.

Osteogenic sarcoma is a children's bone tumor that more closely resembles adult tumors in its resistance to treatment. The most widely used therapy, amputation of the affected limb, has prolonged survival to 5 years in less than 20 percent of patients; more than 50 percent of patients have lung metastases within 5 to 9 months after surgery. In a unique approach based on earlier work by NCI's Goldin and Isaac Djerassi of Mercy Catholic Medical Center in Darby (Philadelphia), Pennsylvania, it has been shown by Norman Jaffe and Emil Frei of the Children's Cancer Research Foundation that metastases can apparently be prevented by massive doses of the antimetabolite methotrexate followed by administration of a compound called citrovorum factor. Methotrexate is an analog of folic acid, a vitamin that is the source of single-carbon fragments in the synthesis of purines for DNA. It inhibits an enzyme called folic acid reductase, and thus impairs replication of malignant and, to a lesser extent, healthy cells. It is one of the most widely used antitumor agents, but it can be used in only limited quantities because of its toxicity to normal cells.

Djerassi has shown, however, that methotrexate can be used in quantities 100 times as great as the normal dose provided that the patient's healthy cells are "rescued" within 6 to 12 hours by citrovorum factor. Citrovorum factor is another folic acid analog that, in essence, substitutes for the normal product of folic acid reductase, thus bypassing the inhibited enzyme. For reasons that are not yet fully understood, this combination of drugs does considerably more damage to malignant cells than to healthy ones. Jaffe's preliminary evidence shows that, of 12 patients treated in this fashion, 11 show no metastases as long as 18 months after amputation.

Some progress in treating osteogenic sarcoma is also being made with other drugs. E. P. Cortes of Queens Hospital Center in New York

City has reported that 14 of 15 patients treated with radical surgery and adriamycin show no evidence of metastases for as much as 26 months after amputation. And Wataru W. Sutow and his associates at M. D. Anderson have reported that 10 of 18 patients treated with a combination of adriamycin, cyclophosphamide, vincristine, and L-sarcolysin have been free of disease for periods of 19 to more than 24 months. Results with Sutow's patients, who have survived the longest of any reported above, indicate that chemotherapy is doing more than simply delaying the onset of metastases.

These data and comparable results with other tumors of children suggest that aggressive chemotherapy which may be only temporarily palliative with a large tumor mass may be curative when there is only a small amount of tumor left after surgery or radiotherapy. Buoyed by their results with the tumors occurring in childhood, investigators are now planning and implementing clinical trials in which multifaceted therapy will be applied to some of the major cancers of adults, including tumors of the breast, lung, and colon. Because recurrences are often naturally delayed for extended periods, however, definitive results will probably not be available for several years.

Another point illustrated by the previously discussed results is the importance of combinations of drugs in treating many types of tumors. Most antitumor agents, as has repeatedly been stressed, have varied side effects associated with their toxicity to healthy cells. Most drugs that interfere with the replication of malignant cells, for example, also kill normal cells that have a high growth fraction—such as cells of the gastrointestinal tract and the bone marrow. These agents thus produce side effects ranging from nausea and hair loss to suppression of the immune system. Adriamycin, a promising antibiotic, causes cardiac problems when the cumulative dose exceeds a certain amount. Vincristine, a vinca alkaloid that halts cell division by destroying the mitotic spindle, is toxic to peripheral nerve cells. And bleomycin, one of the few agents that does not suppress bone marrow, is toxic to lung tissue.

Proper design of combination chemotherapy, says Paul Carbone, involves selection of drugs with both different toxicities and different mechanisms of action. Each drug can then be given in a full dose: The antitumor activities will be additive, but the toxicities to normal cells will not. An additional requirement is that therapy be intermittent so that the normal cells and the immune system may have a chance to recover.

Carbone and DeVita first applied these concepts to Hodgkin's disease when they used a combination of nitrogen mustard, vincristine, procarbazine, and prednisone. This combination, known by the acronym MOPP, more than quadrupled the number of patients who went into complete remission. MOPP has subsequently been adopted by most clinicians for the treatment of Hodgkin's disease, often in combination with radiotherapy. Similar regimens for acute leukemia developed by Frei, Freireich, and Holland have increased the rate of long-term survival in that disease from 0 to more than 50 percent.

Some of the most recent treatment programs can be quite complicated. Norma Wollner and her associates at Memorial Sloan-Kettering, for example, have reported striking results in the treatment of advanced non-Hodgkin's lymphoma with an intricate combination of drugs. Therapy begins with massive doses of cyclophosphamide, followed by radiotherapy to any localized lesions, and a regimen that has also been successfully used in the treatment of acute lymphoblastic leukemia: Vincristine, prednisone, and daunorubicin are given to induce a remission, and are followed by methotrexate to prevent central nervous system involvement, short courses of arabinosylcytosine and thioguanine, twice-weekly doses of L-asparaginase for 4 weeks, a single dose of BCNU [1,3-bis(2-chloroethyl)-1-nitrosourea], and then 6-week cycles of an equally complicated maintenance therapy. Of 35 patients treated with this regimen, 28 still have no evidence of disease after 9 to 34 months. In contrast, 14 of 18 patients previously treated by Wollner with repeated large doses of cyclophosphamide had recurrences of the lymphoma at a median interval of 4 months.

The further application of the concepts developed in the treatment of hemopoietic malignancies and childhood tumors makes the future of chemotherapy against solid tumors look very promising. There are, though, a number of impediments. Perhaps the most important is simply the large number of available agents and the larger number of cancers against which they must be tested. Of the 29 most promising antitumor agents, for example, more than half have been adequately tested in only 4 of the 16 most widely fatal tumors (Table 4). In the remaining 12 major tumors, the percentage that has been tested varies from 17 to 45. There is, moreover, a backlog of promising agents that have never been tested in humans at all. One of the most frequently repeated criticisms of NCI, in fact, is the apparent slow speed at which many potentially curative drugs are moved through the screening and testing processes. Many of these complaints are directed toward the fact that a year or more of toxicological testing must be performed before a new drug can be used in humans; but Zubrod argues that shortcuts in this testing are absolutely inappropriate when the safety of patients is at stake. He further argues that the rate of appearance of new anticancer agents has increased significantly in recent years.

Another problem that has begun to be recognized is an increased incidence of second, apparently unrelated tumors in patients who have been cured of cancer. Of 438 patients treated for Hodgkin's disease at NCI, for example, 14 later developed other types of tumors—a rate that is three to four times the expected incidence for those patients. This increased susceptibility to tumors appears to result from the action of radiation and certain antitumor agents that are thought to be carcinogenic; among patients who received both intensive radiation and suspected drugs, the incidence of second tumors was about 25 times the expected rate.

An alternative explanation is that suppression of the immune system by radiation and antitumor drugs makes the patient more susceptible to other carcinogens. This possibility is supported by recent observations by Israel Penn of the University of Colorado, Boulder, of an increased incidence of tumors among transplant patients who have received immunosuppressive drugs. It has also been shown by Robert A. Good of Memorial Sloan-Kettering that there is an unexpected high incidence of tumors among children with immunodeficiency diseases. In any case, though, it must be remembered that most of the cancer patients in whom the second tumors developed would have been dead long since were it not for the anticancer therapy. The use of potentially carcinogenic therapy thus unquestionably seems justifiable.

A final problem, albeit one that is rapidly disappearing, is the lack of regard for chemotherapists that has historically been exhibited by many surgeons and radiologists. If any one principle has been most firmly demonstrated by recent research in cancer chemotherapy, it is that practitioners from all three disciplines must work together very closely if there is to be a significant improvement in the survival of high-risk patients.

TABLE 4
Availability of Data about Effects of Certain Chemotherapeutic Agents on Selected Tumors
[Source: National Cancer Institute]

Drug	Colon	Lung	Breast	Pancreas	Ovary	Prostate	Stomach	Cervix	Head and neck	Bladder	Kidney	Esophagus	Brain	Testicle	Melanoma	Sarcoma
ALKYLATING AGENTS																
Cytoxan	++	+++	+++	±	+++	±	−	+++	+	±	+	±	+	+++	+	+++
Nitrogen mustard	++	+++	++	−	+	−	−	±	−	−	−	±	+	+++	+	−
Chlorambucil	+	+	++	−	++	−	−	++	−	±	±	−	−	+++	+	++
Melphalan	+	+	+++	−	+++	−	−	+	−	−	−	−	−	+++	+	−
Busulfan	−	+	−	−	−	+	−	−	−	−	−	−	−	−	−	−
ANTIMETABOLITES																
5-Fluorouracil	+++	+	+++	+++	+++	++	++	+++	++	+++	+	+	+	−	+	−
Methotrexate	++	+++	+++	−	−	−	+++	+++	+++	−	−	+	±	−	+	−
6-Mercaptopurine	+	+	+	−	−	−	−	−	−	−	−	−	−	−	+	−
6-Thioguanine	+	−	−	−	−	−	−	−	−	−	−	−	−	−	−	−
Ara-C	+	+	+	−	−	−	−	−	−	−	−	−	−	−	+	−

Mitotic Inhibitors													
Vincristine	+	+	–	+	++	–	++	–	–	–	++	+	+++	–
Vinblastine	+	+	–	+	–	–	–	–	–	–	+	+	+++	–
Antitumor Antibiotics													
Actinomycin D	+	+	–	–	–	–	–	–	–	–	–	++	+++	–
Mithramycin	+	±	–	–	±	–	–	–	–	–	+	±	+++	–
Daunorubicin	–	–	–	–	–	–	–	–	–	–	–	–	–	–
Adriamycin	+	+++	+	++	++	+++	+++	+++	+++	±	++	+++	+++	+++
Bleomycin	+	+	±	+	±	–	++	++	++	–	+++	+++	++	+++
Mitomycin C	+++	++	+	–	+++	++	++	++	–	±	–	++	+++	–
Random Synthetics and Miscellaneous													
BCNU	+++	++	+	++	++	++	–	–	±	±	–	+++	–	–
CCNU	+++	++	–	–	++	++	±	++	–	++	+++	+++	++	–
MeCCNU	+++	++	+	–	++	++	++	–	–	+	++	++	+	–
Streptozotocin	+	+	+	–	–	–	–	–	–	–	–	–	–	–
DTIC	+	+	–	–	++	++	±	–	–	–	++	+++	++	++
Hexamethylmelamine	+	+++	–	++	±	±	+	+	±	–	±	++	–	–
Dibromodulcitol	+	+	–	–	–	++	++	±	±	+	–	+	++	–
Hydroxyurea	+	++	–	–	–	+	–	–	+	±	±	++	++	–
Procarbazine	+	+	–	–	–	–	–	–	–	–	+	+	+	–
L-Asparaginase	+	±	–	–	–	–	–	–	–	–	–	–	–	–
Dibromomannitol	–	–	–	–	–	–	–	–	–	–	–	–	–	–

– = No data; ± = Data barely adequate for some decision on possible activity but without the implication that complete and adequate evaluation of the drug in the tumor has taken place; + = Data adequate to the decision process; ++ = Evidence of clinical activity, although not clearly established; +++ = Definitely established clinical activity.

The search for anticancer drugs is without doubt the largest organized screening program ever undertaken. In the last 20 years, the National Cancer Institute has underwritten the testing of some 300,000 different chemicals to identify the approximately 50 agents that are now either in use or in clinical testing. Rising costs had slowly reduced the number of chemicals tested yearly to about 15,000 only 2 years ago, but the number tested is now up to nearly 50,000 per year. This increase stems, in part, from increased funds made available by the National Cancer Act of 1971. But it has also been made possible by the recent implementation of "mini" and "econo" screens.

The fundamental precept on which the new screens are based is that results with two types of sensitive, transplantable mouse leukemias, called L1210 and P388, are so reliable and reproducible that preliminary screening can be accomplished with far fewer animals. (The L1210 leukemia is used for primary screening of most compounds, but the more sensitive P388 is used for screening natural products.) This screening program, designed primarily by Abraham Goldin and Nathan Mantel of NCI, not only greatly lowers the cost of screening, but also makes it possible to work with much smaller amounts of the chemical to be tested. With the mini screen, for example, it is possible to perform an assay with as little as 3 milligrams of material and as few as 20 mice; the old screening system required a minimum of 65 mg of material and at least 40 mice. Officials at NCI hope that full implementation of the mini and econo screens will at least double the number of chemicals that can be screened for a given amount of money.

A positive result in the preliminary screen is defined as an average 25 percent increase in the life-span of the mice. If a chemical gives a confirmed positive result, as do fewer than 1 out of every 100, it is then tested in mouse lung tumors and skin tumors that are less susceptible to chemotherapeutic agents. A summation of the increased life-spans of mice with the four types of tumors is then used to predict the effect of the drug against human tumors. About 1 of every 1000 agents tested passes this stage. Those that pass, however, must still undergo extensive toxicological and other testing before they can be tried in humans.

The chemicals subjected to the screening procedure can be divided into seven major classes:

1. Compounds that are analogs of known effective agents. A good example is daunorubicin, a glycoside antibiotic that is thought to act by binding to DNA to block its transcription into RNA. Daunorubicin is isolated from *Streptomyces peucetius*, and scientists at the Farmitalia Company in Milan, Italy, found that an artificially produced mutant of this microorganism provides an analog that is hydroxylated at one of its carbon atoms. This analog, adriamycin, is one of the most promising antitumor agents now in use, but it is toxic in that it alters heart action when the cumulative dose exceeds a certain level. Scientists are now looking for analogs of adriamycin that retain the antitumor activity but not the cardiac action.

2. Chemicals developed through biochemical, chemical, cell cycle kinetic, pharmaceutical, and pharmacological concepts. Perhaps the greatest activity in this area involves the search for inhibitors of reverse transcriptase, an enzyme that is crucial to the activity of RNA tumor viruses. This search is proceeding even though viruses have never been shown to cause cancer in humans.

3. Compounds selected from structure-activity relationships. An example of chemicals developed by this approach is the nitrosoureas, such as BCNU, which have proved very effective in treating certain types of tumors.

4. Compounds with new structural features that have not been studied.

5. Compounds showing antitumor activity in programs outside NCI.

6. Compounds isolated from natural sources. Interest in these compounds had died off somewhat as more emphasis was placed on the rational design of antitumor agents, but some scientists feel there has been an upsurge in interest in the last couple of years as the result of the discovery of several promising agents, such as maytansine, an alkaloid isolated and identified by S. Morris Kupchan of the University of Virginia, Charlottesville.

7. Unsolicited compounds from the scientific community at large. The highest priority for testing is given to unstable materials that can be stored for only a short time. Priority is then given, respectively, to compounds found to have clinical activity by outside investigators,

compounds with characteristics superior to those previously tested, compounds developed or acquired at the request of NCI, and all others in the order of receipt.

The successful antitumor agents that have passed through the screen can themselves be divided into at least six classes that reflect their varying mechanisms of action. These classes include the steroidal hormones, alkylating agents, antimetabolites, antibiotics, specific mitotic inhibitors, and miscellaneous drugs.

The era of modern cancer chemotherapy began in the early 1940's when Charles Brenton Huggins of the University of Chicago, Illinois, first used estrogen, one of the *steroidal hormones*, to produce remissions in cancers of the prostate. Other hormones, such as cortisone, prednisone, progesterone, and several androgens, have subsequently been found useful in treatment of some cancers arising from tissues particularly susceptible to hormonal influences. The mechanisms of action of the hormones is not yet understood, but it is possible that they interfere with cell membrane receptors that are involved with the stimulation of growth.

Nitrogen mustard, an *alkylating agent*, was one of the first synthetic chemicals to show antitumor activity. The alkylating agents are generally, but not always, polyfunctional, and are thought to act by cross-linking cellular DNA, thereby impeding its ability to act as a template for RNA synthesis. Other members of this class include chlorambucil, cyclophosphamide, the nitrosoureas, and the imidazole carboximides.

The *antimetabolites* interfere with the biosynthesis of nucleic acids by substituting for normal metabolites in certain enzymic reactions and inhibiting the enzyme. The most important of these are methotrexate, first synthesized by Lederle Laboratories, Pearl River, New York; 5-fluorouracil, synthesized by Charles Heidelberger of the McArdle Laboratory for Cancer Research, Madison, Wisconsin; and 6-mercaptopurine, synthesized by George Hitchings of Burroughs Wellcome Company, Research Triangle Park, North Carolina. More recent members of the class include arabinosylcytosine, thioguanine, and 6-azauridine triacetate.

The *antibiotics* are complex, naturally occurring compounds produced by microbial fermentation. Some, such as daunorubicin, actinomycin D, and adriamycin are thought to bind nonspecifically to cellular

DNA, thus interfering with its transcription. The mechanism of action of others, such as bleomycin and streptozotocin, is not yet known.

The important *mitotic inhibitors* are the vinca alkaloids vincristine and vinblastine. They destroy the mitotic spindle, thereby halting cell division.

The *miscellaneous* drugs do not fall into any of the previous categories. L-Asparaginase, for example, hydrolyzes asparagine in the blood; certain types of tumor cells require an external source of asparagine, and this enzyme blocks that source. Hydroxyurea, while not strictly an antimetabolite, works like one in that it inhibits the enzyme ribonucleoside diphosphate reductase, thus blocking the conversion of cytidylic acid to deoxycytidylic acid, an essential component of DNA. And procarbazine, a methyl hydrazine derivative, depolymerizes cellular DNA.

12
Immunotherapy
New Strategies for Cancer Therapy

The immune system, in the view of many scientists, is the body's principal defense against cancer. It acts in response to antigens present on the surfaces of cancer cells but not on normal cells and destroys the aberrant cells before they can proliferate. Cancer results when a defective immune system fails to perform adequately. If this theory is correct (and possibly even if it isn't), augmenting the body's capacity to mount an immune attack should be a workable strategy for preventing, controlling, or curing cancer.

The current emphasis is on controlling or curing cancer, rather than on preventing it. Although animals have been immunized against cancers, a vaccine for human use will not be available for many years, even by optimistic estimates, because of the numerous technical problems that remain to be solved. Meanwhile, investigators are exploring a number of immunotherapeutic strategies for treating cancer. Some are more advanced in terms of the extent and duration of clinical trials with humans, while others are still in the earliest stages of investigation. All are considered experimental techniques.

The experimental nature of immunotherapy raises bioethical questions for those testing it clinically. No one wants to deprive a cancer patient of the best treatment available. So immunotherapy is often used in conjunction with conventional therapies including chemotherapy—a fact that could complicate interpretation of the results. Alternatively, its use may be restricted to patients who have very poor prognoses, even with the best treatment. They include those suffering from acute myelogenous leukemia, osteogenic sarcoma, or recurrent melanoma, for example, or patients with advanced disease and large tumor burdens. Yet most investigators think that the best application of immunotherapy will be eradication of the relatively few tumor cells remaining after surgery, radiation, or chemotherapy; after such treatment the patient may be clinically free of the disease.

The immune system may be augmented actively if the patient (or his lymphocytes in culture) is directly exposed to stimulating antigens. These can be tumor-associated antigens (active specific immunotherapy), or they can be unrelated to tumor antigens (active nonspecific immunotherapy). The most extensively studied immunotherapies employ BCG (bacillus Calmette-Guérin) and are nonspecific. Bacillus Calmette-Guérin is an attenuated strain of the bacterium that causes bovine tuberculosis. It is frequently used in Europe, and occasionally in the United States, as a vaccine against human tuberculosis. BCG is generally thought to be a potent, nonspecific stimulator of the immune system.

Most data on the use of BCG for cancer therapy derive from studies on patients with melanoma. The primary lesions of melanoma are located in the skin where they are easily accessible for treatment and observation. Among the investigators who have used BCG for treating this cancer are Donald Morton of the University of California Medical Center in Los Angeles and Carl Pinsky and Herbert Oettgen of Memorial Sloan-Kettering Cancer Center in New York City. They found that direct injection of BCG into cutaneous lesions usually causes regression, often complete, of the injected lesions (Figure 23). Sometimes uninjected lesions also regressed. Occasionally, patients treated with BCG have had complete remissions that have lasted for 2 or 3 years or longer. Melanoma, however, despite its usually poor prognosis, is unpredictable and remissions sometimes occur anyway. Metastatic melanoma lesions of the visceral organs or brain are not affected by BCG injections.

Patients with visceral metastases may respond better, however, to a combination of BCG immunotherapy and chemotherapy, according to Jordan Gutterman, Evan Hersh, and their colleagues at M. D. Anderson

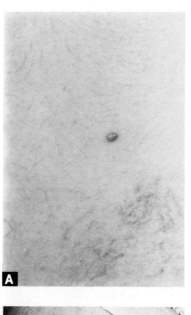

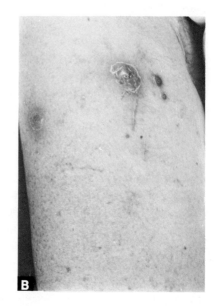

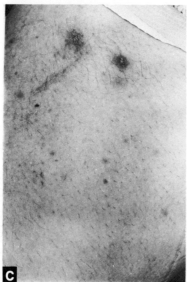

FIGURE 23. Treatment of melanoma metastases with BCG. (A) Close-up view of a melanoma metastasis in skin. (B) Melanoma lesions from the same patient 3 weeks after intralesional injection of BCG. (C) By 4½ months after injection, the melanoma lesions have regressed and the inflammation is subsiding. [Source: Carl Pinsky, Memorial Sloan-Kettering Cancer Center, New York City]

Tumor Institute in Houston, Texas. Their study included 89 patients treated with BCG administered by scarification (the production of superficial scratches into which BCG is introduced) and with the drug dimethyltriazenoimidazole carboxamide (DTIC) and a control group of 111 patients previously treated with DTIC alone. The investigators found that the group receiving the combined therapy survived significantly longer than did the control group. More significantly, they observed prolonged survival of patients with both visceral and nonvisceral metastases, even though the remission rates for patients with visceral metastases was no greater in the study group than in the control group.

The side effects of BCG injection into lesions can be both unpleasant and dangerous. It usually causes inflammation and abscess formation at the injection sites. Pinsky said that more than 40 of the approximately 50 patients in their trial also had fevers lasting several days after the injections. Almost half the patients suffered from recurrent fevers with flulike symptoms, including nausea and vomiting. Liver abnormalities were frequent.

The most dangerous side effect of BCG therapy is a severe hypersensitivity reaction caused by allergy to the organism in individuals who have had more than one exposure. Pinsky had to terminate the BCG therapy of one patient who had a severe reaction. This patient recovered. However, Charles McKhann of the University of Minnesota Medical School, Minneapolis, and Lynn Spitler of the University of California Medical Center in San Francisco, attribute the death of two patients treated with BCG to hypersensitivity to the organism and consequent shock.

There is also the possibility that BCG may depress cell-mediated immunity—the branch of the immune system thought to be most important in fighting cancer—instead of enhancing it. Edmund Klein and his colleagues at Roswell Park Memorial Institute, Buffalo, New York, found that BCG first stimulated the cellular immunity of cancer patients, but continued administration of the agent eventually depressed that immune response in a number of patients. The patients' cellular immunity returned to normal when BCG treatment was discontinued.

Because of these problems, many investigators are exploring the use of other nonspecific stimulators of the immune system that may be less toxic than living BCG. These include membrane fragments and extracts

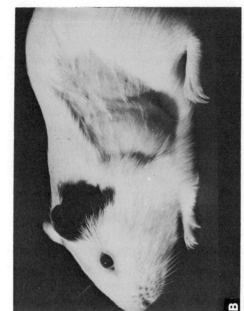

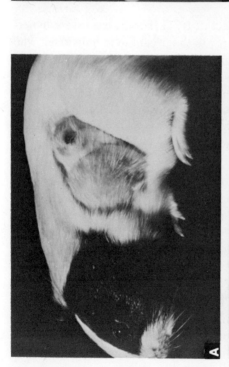

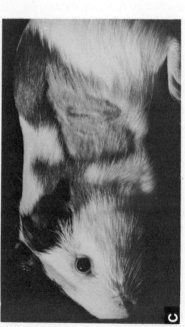

FIGURE 24. Guinea pig model used for investigating immunotherapy. All guinea pigs received an intradermal injection of a highly malignant line of transplantable tumor cells. Six days after injection with tumor cells, the animals received one of three treatments: (A) Diluent used for BCG suspension was injected into the tumor. The tumor (posterior lump) progressed, as did the metastatic tumor in the lymph nodes (anterior lump). The animal died 66 days after inoculation with tumor cells. (B) The tumor was excised. This treatment had no effect on the lymph node metastases, and the animal died 89 days after injection of tumor cells. (C) A preparation of living BCG was injected into the tumor. The tumor regressed, and growth of tumor cells in the lymph nodes was prevented. The animal was still alive 1 year after inoculation with tumor cells. [Source: Herbert Rapp, National Cancer Institute, Bethesda, Maryland]

of BCG, a bacterium called *Corynebacterium parvum*, and a drug named Levamisole. Alternate methods of administering BCG, such as scarification, also produce less severe side effects than does injection into lesions.

Tumor regression induced by BCG may result from the activation of macrophages that attack the tumor cells. Herbert Rapp and Berton Zbar and their colleagues at the National Cancer Institute (NCI), Bethesda, Maryland, have developed a guinea pig model for investigating cancer immunotherapy. Both the immune responses of guinea pigs and the tumors studied (carcinomas) resemble those found in humans.

Rapp and Zbar immunized guinea pigs against one tumor line and then challenged them with intradermal injections of tumor cells. When the challenge cells were from a different line than that used for immunization, tumors grew at the site of injection. When they were from the same line or were a mixture of the two lines, inflammation occurred at the site of injection and tumors did not develop. According to Rapp, tumors did not form at the sites where the mixture was injected because the inflammatory response elicited by tumor cells of the line used for immunization also caused nonspecific destruction of the other tumor cells.

Macrophages appeared to play a role in this nonspecific cell killing. Rapp and Zbar observed large numbers of these cells at the sites of the delayed skin responses. They found that intradermal injection of the macrophages themselves caused inflammation that suppressed the growth of tumor cells subsequently injected into the inflamed sites.

According to Rapp and Zbar, BCG, which produces a strong inflammatory response at the site of injection, suppressed tumor growth when injected with tumor cells. It also induced regression of established tumors and even of early metastatic lesions in the lymph nodes (Figure 24). Larger, more advanced tumors, however, were less susceptible to the effects of BCG. Since Rapp and Zbar, with Michael Hanna of Oak Ridge National Laboratory, Tennessee, observed large numbers of macrophages in the lymph nodes of animals injected with BCG, they hypothesize that the immune system responds to BCG injection with sensitized lymphocytes that can recognize and react with BCG antigens. These lymphocytes then release a product called migration inhibitory factor. Migration inhibitory factor can immobilize macrophages in the injected tumors, where they can destroy tumor cells. Tumor cell destruction releases tumor antigens, which, in turn, provoke additional cell-mediated immune responses, now specific for tumor cells.

There is evidence that macrophages can destroy cancer cells in humans, too. Klein, in collaboration with Isaac Djerassi of Mercy Catholic Medical Center, Darby, Pennsylvania, has used macrophage injections to treat a variety of cancers in humans. The tumors regressed but the treatment is probably not practical for large-scale application. Collection of macrophages is expensive and time-consuming. Furthermore, repeated injections of macrophages may provoke an immune response to the cells themselves, a problem shared with other potential therapies involving injection of cells collected from donors. Nevertheless, the investigators think that their findings constitute further evidence for the importance of macrophages in tumor destruction.

Specific stimulation of the immune system with tumor cells or tumor-associated antigens is another approach to immunotherapy now being explored in a number of laboratories. Much of this work is still in an earlier stage of development than that with BCG. It has been restricted to relatively few human patients and to animal models.

One way of achieving specific activation of a patient's lymphocytes is to culture them with his tumor cells. The sensitized lymphocytes can then be reinfused into the patient where—it is hoped—they will mount an attack on the tumor cells. McKhann has attempted this approach with four patients suffering from widespread metastatic melanoma; only one of the four showed any improvement, and she did not become clinically free of disease.

Another possibility is in vivo stimulation of the immune system by either tumor cells or isolated tumor antigens. Some investigators, such as J. George Bekesi of Mount Sinai School of Medicine, New York City, and Richard Simmons of the University of Minnesota School of Medicine, think that the efficacy of tumor cells in stimulating immune responses can be increased by first treating the cells with the enzyme neuraminidase. This enzyme breaks down the sialic acid coating on the cells; this coat, which is heavier on tumor cells than on normal ones, may mask tumor antigens and thus help the cells escape immune surveillance.

Simmons has found that a number of tumors transplanted into mice regress after injection of tumor cells treated with neuraminidase. The effect is tumor-specific: A tumor will not regress if the treated cells are from a different tumor line. The tumors also failed to regress if the challenge cells had been incubated with neuraminidase inactivated by heating. This indicates that the tumor cells do not provoke an effective immune response unless their antigenicity is increased by the action of the enzyme.

Active specific immunotherapy also increased the survival of mice with spontaneous leukemia, according to Bekesi. If untreated, 95 percent of the animals die within 8 weeks of clinical diagnosis. Immunotherapy with neuraminidase-treated leukemia cells in addition to chemotherapy greatly increased both the percent of animals that survived and the survival time of those that did die when compared to the effects of chemotherapy alone.

Bekesi, with James Holland of Mount Sinai School of Medicine, has begun clinical trials of immunotherapy with neuraminidase-treated leukemia cells for human leukemia. They first reduce the patient's tumor burden to a minimum with chemotherapy. Most investigators think that this step is essential because the immune system has a limited capacity to destroy tumor cells. According to Bekesi, their preliminary results suggest that immunotherapy in addition to chemotherapy increased the length of the patients' remissions by as much as 50 percent over chemotherapy alone. Moreover, when the patients relapsed, additional remissions could more readily be induced.

Immunotherapy can involve a combination of specific and non-specific stimulation of the immune system. For example, Ray Powles and his colleagues at the Chester Beatty Institute in London are using leukemia cells plus BCG to treat adult patients for acute myelogenous leukemia (AML). This leukemia has an extremely poor prognosis; most of the victims die within 1 year of diagnosis. All 53 patients in the study were in complete remission from AML following chemotherapy. Of these, 21 continued on chemotherapy alone while the remaining 32 received both chemotherapy and immunotherapy consisting of weekly injections of irradiated leukemia cells and of BCG. (Tumor cells used in such studies are usually inactivated by irradiation or treatment with inhibitors of cell division in order to avoid the danger of giving tumor cells that are capable of dividing—and producing cancer—to human patients.) Powles found that patients undergoing immunotherapy had longer remissions and survival times than did those who had chemotherapy alone. Immunotherapy did not cure the disease, however.

The immunotherapeutic strategies discussed thus far all involve active stimulation of the patient's immune response. A different way to augment his immune defenses is to transfer specific immune capacity from another individual to the patient. Lymphocytes could be recovered, for example, from a patient cured of a particular cancer and given to another patient afflicted with the same disease. This approach entails major problems. The immune system of the recipient would recognize the lymphocytes as foreign and destroy them. Severe hypersensitivity reactions, like those occasionally observed with BCG, might also occur.

Use of whole cells may be unnecessary, however. Recent research suggests that certain products of the immune system can transfer specific immunity between individuals without themselves evoking undesirable immune responses. The two such products receiving the widest attention are transfer factor and immune RNA.

Transfer factor, which was discovered by H. Sherwood Lawrence of New York University School of Medicine, New York City, about 20 years ago, transfers cell-mediated immunity from one individual to another, possibly by activating the recipient's lymphocytes. The material is isolated from lymphocytes. It is a conjugate of nucleic acid (probably RNA) and polypeptide. Since transfer factor has a molecular weight of less than 10,000, it is not immunogenic.

Because of these properties, investigators think that transfer factor may be useful for cancer therapy. It is especially important that it transfers cell-mediated, but not humoral, immunity/ Blocking factor, which can prevent the attack of lymphocytes on tumor cells, may be a complex of antibody with tumor antigens. Stimulation of humoral immunity—and antibody production—could increase the blocking activity in a cancer patient's serum and thus interfere with his response to immunotherapy or even enhance tumor growth. This is a potential problem with any therapy in which the immune system is stimulated, but it should not be a deterrent to the use of transfer factor.

Although many investigators think that transfer factor is specific—eliciting immune responses in the recipient only to those antigens to which the donor can respond—this has not yet been definitively established and is a matter of some dispute. Nevertheless, transfer factor for cancer therapy is often prepared from the lymphocytes of people who can be shown to have immunity to antigens associated with the tumor in question. Since evidence indicates that tumors of the same type have common antigens, the donors could be individuals cured of the particular cancer. They could also be members of the patient's immediate family or very close associates.

Morton has shown that relatives of patients suffering from osteogenic sarcoma have a much higher incidence of antibodies to the tumor than do members of the general population. Alan Levin, working with H. Hugh Fudenberg at the University of California Medical Center in San Francisco, has shown that more than 20 percent of the household contacts of individuals with osteogenic sarcoma have strong cell-mediated immunity to the tumor. These results imply—but do not prove—that a virus causes this cancer. Only a few of those exposed to the putative virus get the disease, presumably because of their failure to mount an effective immune response.

The prognosis of osteogenic sarcoma, a bone cancer affecting children primarily, is dismal: Approximately 80 percent of the victims develop metastases in the lungs within 6 months of diagnosis even though the primary lesion is removed surgically. Levin and Fudenberg have so far used transfer factor in the treatment of 12 patients with osteogenic sarcoma. Two have died and two have been switched to chemotherapy, but the remaining eight have been tumor-free and without metastases for up to 18 months.

According to Levin and Fudenberg, treatment with transfer factor is not suitable for patients who already have more than one pulmonary metastasis. It causes inflammation of those lesions that may itself threaten the patient's life. As with other immunotherapies, transfer factor should be most valuable for killing residual tumor cells and preventing metastasis after successful removal of the primary tumor. Another problem is the possible depletion of the donor's capacity to mount an immune response to tumor antigens. Fudenberg has evidence that this happens after extensive removal of the donor's lymphocytes. The donors recovered the capacity after the lymphocyte collections were halted, but this finding raises the question of whether it is safe to deprive humans—especially cured cancer patients—of their immune defenses against cancer. Despite these problems, results from Fudenberg's laboratory and from a number of others are encouraging investigators to undertake more extensive, controlled experiments with transfer factor for cancer therapy.

Immune RNA is another substance that can be used to transfer cell-mediated immunity between individuals, according to Yosef Pilch of the University of California School of Medicine, Los Angeles. Pilch has shown that immune RNA, which is extracted from lymphoid tissues, can elicit immune responses against tumors both in vivo and in vitro. The effects were specific for the type of tumor used to immunize the donors of immune RNA but they were not species-specific. For example, immune RNA extracted from the lymphoid organs of guinea pigs that had been immunized against a rat tumor protected rats against the growth of transplants of the tumor.

Pilch has extracted immune RNA from the lymphocytes of humans cured of melanoma. The RNA could convert normal human lymphocytes to cells cytotoxic to cultured melanoma cells. Moreover, immune RNA extracted from lymphoid cells of sheep that had been immunized to a human melanoma doubled the cytotoxic activity of the human patient's lymphocytes against his own melanoma cells in culture.

As long as immune RNA is free of protein contamination, it is weakly antigenic, if at all, and is well tolerated by patients. This property, in conjunction with the ability to use animal rather than human donors and the tumor specificity of immune RNA, makes its potential use for cancer immunotherapy an attractive prospect.

At present there is insufficient data to evaluate and compare immunotherapeutic strategies with each other and with conventional therapies. There have been promising results, especially in treating patients with accessible tumors including melanoma and other skin cancers, but only if there are no internal metastases. Other data indicate that the capacity of the immune system to control tumor growth is limited, and many investigators think that immunotherapy must be restricted to patients whose tumor burdens have already been reduced to very low levels by conventional techniques.

There are unanswered questions and unsolved problems concerning potential hazards of immunotherapy. These include hypersensitivity reactions and the possibility of evoking an autoimmune response in which the patient's immune system attacks his normal tissues instead of just tumor cells. This could happen if the antigens used to stimulate the immune system were found on normal cells and not just on tumor cells. Stimulation of the immune system might also result in increased production of blocking factors and enhanced tumor growth. Investigators think that intensive monitoring of the patient's immune responses with in vivo and in vitro assays is required for assessing the efficacy of immunotherapies.

Other therapies in addition to those described here are being considered. Only time—and careful, well-controlled clinical trials—will tell which are most satisfactory for cancer therapy.

13
After Cancer Therapy
Rehabilitating the Patient

Most people dread cancer more than any other disease. Their fear cannot be attributed only to fear of death. After all, heart disease claims twice as many victims as cancer does. But people usually associate cancer with radical, disfiguring treatments, consequent disability, and then a lingering and painful death. In other words, the popular view is that cancer not only destroys life but also destroys the quality and usefulness of whatever life remains after diagnosis and therapy.

This is a portrait of cancer at its worst. But there is growing recognition that it is a picture which is far too pessimistic. According to figures compiled by the National Cancer Institute (NCI) in Bethesda, Maryland, there are 1.5 million people in the United States whose cancers have been cured or controlled, as judged by their survival for 5 or more years after diagnosis. Moreover, this number is constantly growing. More than one-third of the approximately 655,000 new cases of cancer diagnosed each year will be added to the cured or controlled group. In comprehensive cancer centers the percentage of patients whose cancers are cured or controlled may be even higher, approaching 45 to 50 percent, so as advanced or experimental therapies become more widely accepted, the overall cure rate should increase.

Early diagnosis also increases the likelihood of a favorable prognosis. For example, if cancer of the colon or breast is treated before it spreads to the lymph nodes, 80 percent or more of the patients live at least 5 years, but that number drops to 30 to 40 percent if the cancer has spread. Since fear and pessimism contribute to a person's reluctance to seek early treatment, many clinicians think that there should be greater emphasis, both within and without the medical profession, on successes in cancer therapy rather than on the failures.

Widespread availability of rehabilitative services may also help allay a person's fears. Even cured patients may be left with disfigurements, disabilities, or psychological handicaps that prevent them from resuming their normal lives. Patients with poor prognoses may have similar handicaps plus the emotional need to cope with the imminence of their own deaths. So there is a growing trend toward developing and providing the rehabilitative or supportive services that cancer patients need to live the fullest lives possible. In fact, the seventh and last objective specified by the National Cancer Act of 1971 is: "Develop the means to improve the rehabilitation of cancer patients."

What does rehabilitation mean? Lawrence Burke, program director for rehabilitation of the Treatment, Rehabilitation, and Continuing Care Branch at NCI, subdivides it into three components:

1. Physical restoration of defects such as those caused by surgery to remove a cancerous organ or body part. Patients treated for different cancers will, of course, have different problems. Some will need artificial limbs; others, plastic surgery or prosthetic devices to replace facial parts; still others, training in the management of stomas (artificial body openings) such as those created by removal of the larynx or of the colon, rectum, or bladder. All may need training in order to live with residual defects.

2. Psychosocial counseling to enable the patient to cope with the emotional impact of cancer, including fear of recurrence of the disease and death, and to adjust to any disfigurement.

3. Vocational training, if necessary, in order that the patient may once again be self-sufficient and not dependent on family assistance or the welfare agency. This includes training the housewife to perform as much as possible of her normal work as well as retraining the wage-earner who may no longer be able to perform his or her former job.

The multifaceted requirements of the cancer patient cannot be met by any one person, according to John E. Healey, Jr., former head of the department of Rehabilitation Medicine at M. D. Anderson Hospital and Tumor Institute in Houston, Texas, and now associate director of the Division of Cancer Control at the University of Miami Comprehensive Cancer Center in Florida. The attending physician may need to call on a variety of professionals with expertise in different areas. This need is reflected in the team approach to rehabilitation utilized at cancer centers such as M. D. Anderson and Memorial Sloan-Kettering Cancer Center in New York City.

Although the participation of individual members may vary depending on the needs of a given patient, the team described by J. Herbert Dietz, Jr., of Memorial Hospital for Cancer and Allied Diseases, New York City, is typical of those recommended for comprehensive cancer centers. It includes the attending physician who has the primary responsibility for the patient's treatment, a physician specializing in rehabilitation medicine, the nurse who assists the team and helps the patient to learn self-care techniques, physical and occupational therapists, a social worker, a psychiatrist or clinical psychologist, and appropriate consultants.

Some hospitals do not have enough cancer patients to justify employing all of these professionals. Burke says that, in addition to sponsoring demonstration facilities such as those at comprehensive cancer centers, NCI plans to encourage smaller hospitals to coordinate their facilities so that the needed services would be available within a given area or community even if not within the walls of one institution.

The history of coordinated efforts to rehabilitate cancer patients is short—only about 10 years. Among the pioneering rehabilitation programs are those at M. D. Anderson and Memorial Sloan-Kettering. The latter originated as a cooperative venture between the Institute of Rehabilitation Medicine of New York University Medical Center and Memorial Hospital for Cancer and Allied Diseases; it is now wholly based at Memorial Sloan-Kettering. Similar services are offered at a number of other cancer centers including those at Roswell Park Memorial Institute in Buffalo, New York, the University of Washington Medical School in Seattle, the University of Alabama School of Medicine in Birmingham, and, most recently, the University of Texas Health Science Center in Dallas.

The late recognition of the need of the cancer patient for rehabilitation and the lack of interest in, or even resistance to, this subject that persist even today can be attributed to a number of factors, according to Dietz, Healey, and others. Not the least of these is the widespread pessimism about the fate of individuals suffering from the disease. Although the picture is changing, this pessimism has existed in all sectors of the population, including the medical profession and the government agencies that might support rehabilitative services.

At one time, rehabilitative aid was not offered to the patient until he had been free of cancer for 12 to 18 months. At best this delayed and hindered a person's return to a full life, and at worst deprived him virtually all the useful time left to him. The current trend is to begin rehabilitation immediately—as soon as the disability can be predicted. For example, a person whose leg is going to be amputated learns to walk with crutches before the operation, while his balance is good and before muscles deteriorate from disuse. He is then fitted with an artificial leg immediately after surgery.

There has also been a shortage of personnel willing to work with cancer patients. Medical personnel, whether physicians, nurses, or other paramedical professionals, do not like to be confronted with their own vulnerability, mortality, or fallibility any more than anyone else does—and possibly less than others do. The American Cancer Society (ACS) and NCI are now sponsoring training programs for technicians, such as enterostomal therapists, who will work with cancer patients. According to Healey, physicians may have received an overly pessimistic view of cancer during medical training, when the few patients they encountered in the hospital were advanced or terminal cases.

Another reason for the lack of rehabilitative services is that the American medical system has been mostly concerned with acute care—curing or controlling the disease and then sending the patient home. Except for periodic examinations to check for recurrence of the cancer, there was little concern about how well the individual fared in his family, social, and vocational life after dismissal from the hospital.

Even now there is a dearth of information about the quality of a person's life after treatment for cancer. Dietz says, however, that up to 95 percent of all cancer patients can benefit from rehabilitative services. The goals for each patient depend on his prognosis and physical capabilities.

They are restorative if the patient can be expected to function as he did before the onset of the disease and with little or no residual handicap; supportive if the disease or handicap will persist but training and treatment can eliminate as much of the handicap as possible; or palliative if progressing disease will produce further disability but appropriate treatment can eliminate some of the complications that might otherwise ensue.

Of approximately 1000 patients referred for rehabilitative services to Memorial Hospital every year, Dietz estimates that almost 10 percent achieve full recovery; up to 30 percent show marked improvement in spite of residual disability; 40 percent respond satisfactorily with lessened disability but with persistent disease; and only about 20 percent show no improvement. As might be expected, those in the restorative group had the greatest success in achieving their goals and those in the palliative group the least. Dietz says that the rehabilitation team may push an individual with a good prognosis harder than one whose prognosis is poor to prevent him from falling into unnecessary dependency. Patients with poor prognoses are not subjected to unnecessary stress.

The limited data available indicate that the potential for vocational rehabilitation of cancer patients is comparable to that of people suffering from other chronic diseases. Healey says that data from the Texas Division of Vocational Rehabilitation (DVR) showed that 29.5 percent of the 142 cancer patients assisted during fiscal year 1967–1968 achieved vocational rehabilitation (as measured by their returning to gainful employment or regaining independence from the assistance of family members or welfare agencies).

This rate was higher than that for people with diseases such as heart disease (15.3 percent rehabilitated), diabetes (13.4 percent), and orthopedic deformities (10.5 percent). Moreover, the cost of rehabilitating cancer patients was lower than that for other patients. Yet the number of cancer patients aided by the DVR was very low. This is still an improvement over the earlier situation, however. Until 1966, the Department of Health, Education, and Welfare provided extremely limited funds for the vocational rehabilitation of cancer patients.

In order to fill the vacuum resulting from the earlier neglect of rehabilitation, the patients developed their own programs for aiding others who suffered the same handicaps. Perhaps the best known of these is the Reach to Recovery program. This was started in the early 1950's by Terese Lasser after she had a mastectomy and discovered how little assistance was available for helping women adjust to the aftereffects of this operation.

Since 1969, the ACS has sponsored Reach to Recovery. William Markel, Vice President for Service and Rehabilitation of the ACS, says that the program has 6000 volunteers—all women who are trained by the ACS to give the appropriate psychological support to a patient who may be both frightened by her disease and insecure about her image as a woman after removal of a breast.

The volunteers visit the patient, only if requested by her physician, a few days after her surgery while she is still in the hospital. They provide information about obtaining prosthetic devices and about finding and fitting attractive clothing. They also give the woman a Reach to Recovery kit containing a breast form, simple exercise equipment, and directions for doing exercises to help the patient regain full movement of her arm and shoulder. (During most mastectomy operations, the muscles of the chest and under the arm may be removed and the scar itself may inhibit motion.) Markel says that during fiscal year 1972–1973, the volunteers made 32,000 such visits—which means that they saw more than half of the mastectomy patients during that period.

The International Association of Laryngectomees and the United Ostomy Association sponsor clubs and offer moral support as well as practical advice to persons who have had their larynxes removed or who have stomas. Both organizations are affiliated with the ACS but not controlled by it, and both include people who have had their operations for reasons other than cancer.

The clinicians interviewed say that cancer patients do not receive rehabilitative services unless they are requested by the attending physician. (Two exceptions are found at Memorial Hospital, where patients who have had mastectomies or thoracic surgery are automatically enrolled in classes at the hospital that aim to teach them to cope with and overcome their disabilities.) They point out that physicians and patients alike need to be educated about the kinds of services that are available and motivated to use them. In some cases, where the attending physician resists "interference" from third parties, the patient or the patient's family requires the knowledge—and the stamina—to provide the impetus toward rehabilitation.

Finally, the clinicians say that cancer needs a new image. It is not the invariably debilitating killer it once was, and, when properly treated, a third or more of the victims have a normal life expectancy. All cancer patients have a right to live as full lives as possible for as long as possible.

IV
Specific Cancers

14

The Organ Site Approach to Cancer Research

Cancers of the colon and rectum, breast, lung, prostate, and bladder accounted for more than 50 percent of the new cancers detected during 1974, according to estimates compiled by the National Cancer Institute (NCI) in Bethesda, Maryland (Table 5). Because of their importance as health hazards, these cancers are the targets of the first five organ site programs established by NCI. The purpose of the programs is the accumulation and application of knowledge needed to prevent the occurrence of specific cancers and to improve the survival rates of persons who do contract them.

Task forces have been established by NCI to coordinate research on breast, bladder, prostate, and colorectal cancers. There is no current lung cancer task force, although one did exist at an earlier time. The responsibility for lung cancer research is now split between such groups as the Tobacco Working Group (a contract review committee advisory to NCI) and the Lung Cancer Branch in the Division of Cancer Cause and Prevention at NCI.

The breast cancer task force (BCTF), headed by Nathaniel Berlin of NCI, is the oldest—established in 1967—of the organ site coordinating

TABLE 5

Estimated Number of New Cases and Deaths for Selected Cancers, 1974
[Source: National Cancer Institute]

Cancer site	Estimated new cases in 1974	Estimated deaths in 1974
Colon and rectum	99,000	48,000
Breast	90,000	33,000
Lung	83,000	75,000
Prostate	54,000	18,000
Head and neck		
Oral	23,700	7900
Larynx	10,000	3000
Bladder	28,400	9200
Pancreas	20,300	19,400

groups. The other three task forces have been established since passage of the National Cancer Act in 1971. According to David Joftes of the National Organ Site Programs Branch (this branch of the Division of Cancer Research Resources and Centers oversees the bladder, prostate, and large bowel organ site projects but not those concerned with breast and lung cancer), there are also plans to initiate task forces to tackle cancer of the pancreas and of the head and neck. The former disease is particularly interesting because the incidence of pancreatic cancer has been steadily increasing—for unknown reasons—for several years. This cancer has an especially poor prognosis: The 5-year survival rate is only about 1 or 2 percent.

All research done under the aegis of the task forces is targeted—directed at achieving specific goals—but there are differences in the ways the task forces operate. The BCTF funds virtually all its research by contracts whereas the other three task forces fund theirs by grants. (Most lung cancer research is also funded by contracts.) Another difference is that the leadership of the BCTF is located at NCI. The headquarters of the bladder, large bowel, and prostate task forces are located at institutions outside of NCI: the bladder task force at St. Vincent Hospital, Worcester, Massachusetts, under the direction of Gilbert Friedell; the large bowel task force at M. D. Anderson Hospital and Tumor Institute, Houston, Texas, under the direction of Murray Copeland; and the prostate task force at Roswell Park Memorial Institute, Buffalo, New York, under the direction of Gerald Murphy.

Establishment of the headquarters of these task forces at institutions other than NCI and their use of the grant rather than the contract mechanism for funding research has apparently been in response to some of the criticisms leveled at NCI's management of cancer research. One of these criticisms concerns the possibility that research programs directed centrally from NCI may become too rigid—resulting in rejection of otherwise meritorious research proposals that do not fit the NCI plan and in inability to respond to unexpected research results. Another is that contracts may be awarded without rigorous enough scrutiny of the applications for their scientific merit.

Grant applications submitted to any institute of the National Institutes of Health (NIH) are generally reviewed by study groups, composed of nongovernment scientists, that approve or disapprove the applications on the basis of their scientific merit and assign them a priority rating for the available money. The appropriate institute and its advisory board then decides which of the approved grants will actually be funded. While applications for grants are submitted at the initiative of the investigator and, theoretically at least, without regard for their practical value, applications for contracts are submitted in response to a specific Request for Proposals (RFP) issued by the contracting agency. The RFP specifies a particular goal to be achieved and may also specify the approach to be taken in reaching it. The contract review committees consist of a mix of both government and nongovernment scientists, but some investigators who have served on them claim that the government scientists have a disproportionate amount of influence over the decisions.

According to Joftes and the task force directors, the bladder, large bowel, and prostate task forces are composed entirely of nongovernment scientists and function more like traditional study groups. A difference is that the task forces consider whether a proposal is relevant to the goals they have established in addition to evaluating its scientific merit. Potential for practical application is not a concern for many of the fifty or so study sections that review grant proposals for NIH. Although these three task forces have set goals and drawn up plans, Joftes says that the grant mechanism is more flexible in permitting consideration of proposals involving approaches or concepts that are not specified in a plan but are both meritorious and relevant.

Despite these mechanical differences, the scientific strategies of the four task forces are similar. Their approach as exemplified by the BCTF, which is understandably the most advanced, includes the following main topics of interest: determining the cause or causes of the cancer (epidemiology and etiology); seeking ways to prevent development of the disease in individuals at risk because of their exposure to environmental carcinogens; developing techniques that can detect the cancers in the early stages; and improving the treatment and survival rate of those who do develop the disease. Despite the emphasis on applied research, there is room in the organ site programs for basic studies of the biology of normal and cancerous organs.

The trend toward targeted research displayed by NCI in the past few years has, however, been the subject of considerable controversy in the scientific community. The assumption underlying the trend is that there is enough basic knowledge about the activities of normal and cancer cells and the differences between them to allow selection of appropriate goals and solution of whatever problems must be solved to achieve those goals. This assumption has itself been the target of frequent criticism, especially from investigators engaged in basic research, but many scientists at NCI think that targeted research will in fact pay off. They also argue that central direction can better coordinate research in diverse areas and result in improved health care for the public—a worthwhile goal since it is the public that pays for the research. None of these controversies will be easily resolved, but then neither will the cancer problem.

15
Breast Cancer Research

Problems and Progress

Breast cancer is the third most prevalent type of cancer in the United States, according to figures compiled by the National Cancer Institute (NCI) in Bethesda, Maryland. An estimated 90,000 new cases of, and 33,000 deaths from, this disease occurred in 1974. The fact that the breast cancer death rate has remained essentially constant for the last 35 years provides a stimulus for ongoing research into the causes, detection, and treatment of the disease. Although fundamental questions remain unanswered, investigators are encouraged by recent developments, especially in the areas of detection and chemotherapy.

Much of the breast cancer research is performed under the aegis of the breast cancer task force (BCTF) of NCI. The BCTF program is the oldest (established in 1966) and most extensively funded ($7.1 million in fiscal year 1974) of the organ site projects of NCI. These projects are directed at gathering and applying the information necessary for improving the survival of patients with a specific cancer. Virtually all research sponsored by the BCTF is targeted—intended to achieve specific research goals—and funded by contracts.

Since more than 99 percent of breast cancer victims are women, it is estimated that one woman of every 15 will develop the disease sometime in her lifetime. One of the research goals is the identification of women who are at greatest risk from breast cancer. Epidemiological studies have identified a number of risk indicators. As with other cancers, several biological, environmental, genetic—and, possibly, viral—factors appear to interact in the etiology of breast cancer.

The incidence of breast cancer is five to six times higher in North America and northern Europe than it is in most of Asia and Africa. Among the explanations advanced to account for these geographic variations are differences in genetic and environmental factors, including diet. In high-risk areas the incidence increases with age. Although there is a plateau or even a dip in the incidence curve at about the age of menopause, breast cancer, like most other cancers, is primarily a disease of old age.

Breast cancer appears to run in families. According to figures supplied by the American Cancer Society (ACS), daughters and sisters of breast cancer patients are two to three times more likely to develop the disease than are women not related to breast cancer patients. David Anderson of M. D. Anderson Hospital and Tumor Institute in Houston, Texas, found that the risks were even higher—six to nine times the general risk—if the patient's disease occurred before menopause and involved both breasts. As with most other situations of this type, both heredity and environment could be involved, and sorting out their relative influences is difficult.

A woman's reproductive history is one of the biological factors that determine her chances of developing breast cancer. According to Brian MacMahon of the Harvard School of Public Health, Boston, Massachusetts, the risk increases with the age at which she has her first full-term pregnancy. Pregnancy before age 30 is protective in the sense that these women are less likely to develop breast cancer than are women who have never had a child. Only a full-term pregnancy confers protection. Having a first child after 30 increases the risk compared to that of nulliparous women. Neither lactation nor additional pregnancies, after the first, have significant effects on the incidence of the disease. Although no one knows the mechanism by which reproductive history influences susceptibility to breast cancer, the female sex hormones are probably involved.

Other evidence has also implicated these hormones in mammary carcinogenesis. MacMahon and others have found that both early onset and late cessation of menstruation are associated with an increased risk of breast cancer. Menstruation, of course, depends on the production of the ovarian hormones estrogen and progesterone. Although estrogens especially are known to stimulate the division of sensitive cells—and cancer is characterized by uncontrolled cell division—the exact role of hormones in breast cancer etiology is unclear.

A question frequently raised in conjunction with the relationship between hormones and breast cancer is what effect—if any—contraceptive pills have on the risk of developing the disease. According to Heinz Berendes of the Center for Population Research of the National Institute of Child Health and Human Development, none of the studies conducted thus far show any association between contraceptive pills, most of which contain both estrogens and progesterones, and breast cancer. Most of the studies have been retrospective, but one recent prospective study, conducted by Clifford R. Kay for the Royal College of General Practitioners in Great Britain, also showed no correlation. Nevertheless, Berendes points out that the results of these studies must be interpreted cautiously. The "pill" has been in widespread use for less than 10 years whereas the estimated time period required for the development of most cancers, including breast cancer, is 15 to 20 years.

In addition to the ovarian hormones, those of the adrenal and pituitary glands have been implicated in mammary oncogenesis. Recently, attention has been focused on prolactin, a hormone secreted by the pituitary gland and required for lactation. Evidence acquired by Clifford Welsch of the College of Human Medicine, Michigan State University, East Lansing, indicates that this hormone may be essential for breast cancer development in mice and rats. Welsch also found that addition of prolactin to cultures of malignant human breast tissue stimulated growth of the tissues. A number of investigators are exploring the role of prolactin in the growth and maintenance of human breast cancers.

Viruses play a prominent role in any discussion of the etiology of breast cancer. They have been known as a cause of mammary cancer in mice since 1936 when the Bittner or mouse mammary tumor virus (MMTV) was discovered. The MMTV is an RNA virus of type B.

Many investigators think that a similar virus is involved in the etiology of human mammary cancer. Although their evidence indicates that such a virus may exist, definitive proof remains elusive—just as it does for all viruses implicated in the etiology of human cancers.

Human milk may be one source of viral particles. For example, Dan Moore and his colleagues at the Institute for Medical Research, Camden, New Jersey, observed particles with the morphological properties of type B viruses in electron micrographs of human milk samples. The presence of the particles did not, however, correlate with the donor's family history of breast cancer.

Substances present in human milk can destroy virus particles. Moore and others have found that human milk causes the breakdown of MMTV. The mechanism of virus damage is not yet known, but it undoubtedly interferes with attempts to detect virus particles by electron microscopy.

Biochemical evidence also indicates the presence of oncogenic RNA viruses (oncornaviruses) in human milk. Such viruses are characterized by their density (1.16 to 1.19 grams per milliliter), by the presence of $60S$ to $70S$ RNA (S is the symbol for the Svedberg unit, a measure of the rate at which a material sediments in the ultracentrifuge), and by the presence of the enzyme reverse transcriptase. This enzyme synthesizes DNA copies of viral RNA and is necessary for the function of oncogenic RNA viruses. Sol Spiegelman of the Columbia University College of Physicians and Surgeons, New York City, and Jeffrey Schlom, now at NCI, with Moore, found particles with these properties in human milk samples.

In addition to substances that destroy virus particles, human milk contains the enzyme ribonuclease, according to Marvin Rich, Michael Brennan, and their colleagues at the Michigan Cancer Foundation, Detroit. This enzyme interferes with biochemical tests for oncorna-viruses, which depend on determining the activity of reverse transcrip-tase, because it destroys the RNA template needed for DNA synthesis. Rich said that reverse transcriptase can still be detected if its concentration is high as compared to that of ribonuclease. Nevertheless, the presence in human milk of these interfering substances has complicated attempts to correlate the presence of virus particles with risk of contracting breast cancer.

The presence of particles resembling known oncogenic RNA viruses in human milk does not prove that these particles are involved in the etiology of human cancer. There is no evidence that human mammary cancer is transmitted, as it is in certain strains of mice, by an agent in milk. In fact, although breast-feeding has declined dramatically in the United States in the last 50 to 60 years, the incidence of breast cancer has not decreased and may have increased slightly.

Other evidence implicating viruses in the etiology of breast cancer does not depend on the use of human milk. Spiegelman and Schlom used reverse transcriptase to synthesize DNA complementary to MMTV. They showed that 66 percent of 29 human breast tumors contained RNA that hybridized with this DNA. This indicated that the tumor RNA is itself complementary to the DNA and must therefore have base sequences and information content similar to that of a known oncogenic virus.

Rich and his colleagues found a virus with the characteristics of an oncornavirus replicating in a line of cultured cells derived from a patient with carcinoma of the breast. The cultured cells are of human epithelial origin. (Carcinomas are cancers of epithelial cells.) They have certain properties of mammary cells, including the presence of receptors that bind estrogen and the ability to synthesize lactalbumin. Rich says that the evidence strongly suggests that the virus is of human origin.

The relationship of this virus to the particles found in human milk and to the etiology of human breast cancer is under investigation. Because of the dismal history of some other human cancer virus candidates that have come—and then quickly gone—the investigators are understandably cautious about the meaning of their findings. In any event, a virus caught at the scene of the crime is not necessarily the culprit.

Most investigators think that viruses, if they are involved at all, are necessary but not sufficient causes of mammary carcinogenesis. If they are necessary, then preventive measures based on interference with viral function may be possible. Moore and his colleagues can prevent mammary tumors in mice with a vaccine made from killed MMTV. Such a vaccine is not feasible for human use because it requires administration of nucleic acid from an oncogenic virus. A vaccine for human use would have to contain only such viral constituents as proteins or glycoproteins. A different preventive strategy, the use of drugs to inhibit viral expression or the activity of reverse transcriptase, is under investigation in a number of laboratories.

Until prevention of cancer becomes a reality, control of breast cancer requires that it be detected and then treated successfully. As with other types of cancer, early detection—before the cancer metastasizes to other parts of the body—is thought to be a prerequisite for successful treatment. Sixty percent of breast cancer patients live for 5 years after their disease is diagnosed. But large differences in survival are apparent between patients with localized disease and those with disseminated disease—80 percent of the former live 5 years or longer whereas only 45 percent of the latter do. Thus, many clinicians think that screening (periodic examinations of large numbers of apparently healthy women by trained personnel) might increase the detection of early breast cancers—and improve the survival rate.

One of the largest studies conducted thus far showed that mass screening by clinical examination or manual palpation of the breasts, in conjunction with mammography, can reduce the mortality from breast cancer. Mammography is low-voltage x-ray examination of the breast, with the image recorded on conventional x-ray film. The study, conducted by Philip Strax of the New York Medical College, New York City, began in 1963 and includes 62,000 women between the ages of 40 and 64 years. The women, who are members of the Health Insurance Plan of Greater New York, were selected as 31,000 matched pairs, one set of which was the study group and the other the control group. Of the study group, 65 percent agreed to be screened for breast cancer and to have three subsequent annual check-ups.

According to Strax, the death rate of the study group from breast cancer was one-third lower than that of the control group after 5 years. Seventy percent of the patients whose cancers were detected by screening were free of metastases. The comparable figure for the control group was 46 percent. Moreover, the study demonstrated the utility of mammography in screening: 44 cancers (33 percent of the total) not found by palpation were detected by the x-ray technique. Strax said that only one of the 44 women whose cancers were detected by mammography alone has died of her cancer. On the other hand, 59 cancers not found by mammography were detected by clinical examination. Thus, both techniques contributed to detection of the cancers.

One of the disadvantages of mammography for periodic screening of healthy women is that x-rays are themselves carcinogenic. Use of fast x-ray film has decreased the radiation dose to about 1 to 2 rads (a rad is a measure of the radiation energy absorbed by exposed material) per exposure. Variations of mammography, such as xeroradiography (Figure 25), in which a different system is used for recording the x-ray image, also permit a lower radiation dose than do older mammographic techniques.

Thermography entails no radiation at all. Instead, an infrared detector is used to produce a photograph of the skin's heat pattern. Cancers are indicated by the presence of "hot spots" due either to the altered metabolism of the tumor or to its increased blood supply (Figure 26). Thermography is not specific for cancer because other, benign, conditions may also produce such hot spots. But it can be used for screening with additional tests used as necessary to confirm the diagnosis.

The ACS sponsored a collaborative pilot study involving several medical centers to evaluate the potential of thermography in cancer detection. The results of the study showed that thermography detects cancers not found by palpation in addition to some not detectable by mammography. Thus, each of the three techniques in greatest use—palpation, mammography, and thermography—detects different groups of cancers. The ACS and NCI now sponsor 27 breast cancer detection centers where women can obtain free examinations. All three techniques are used at the centers, and breast self-examination is also taught. At each of these centers, at least 5000 women will be examined every year. There are, however, approximately 40 million women over 40 in the United States. Although both NCI and the ACS stress the importance of early detection, monetary and personnel limitations prohibit extension of screening to all of them.

Once localized breast cancer is detected, the primary treatment is surgery, sometimes accompanied by radiation therapy. Cancers too extensive to remove surgically are usually treated with radiation or chemotherapy and often by removal of one or more of the three glands—ovaries, adrenals, and pituitary—known to influence tumor growth. The therapies for advanced disease are palliative, not curative.

For many years, a controversy has raged over how extensive the surgery must be for successful treatment of breast cancer. The Halsted radical mastectomy, the most commonly used operation, entails removal

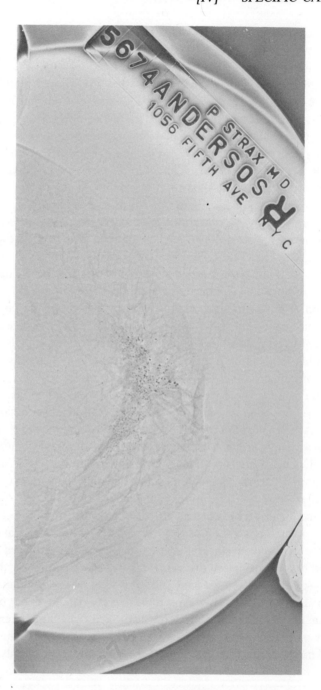

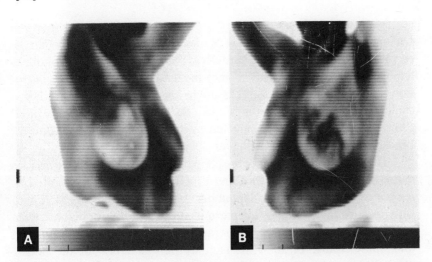

FIGURE 26. Thermograms of a normal breast (A) and a cancerous breast (B). Areas of increased temperature, which may be due to a malignant tumor, are darker than areas with lower temperatures. [Source: Philip Strax, Guttman Institute, New York City]

of the entire breast, the underlying chest muscles, and the lymph nodes in the axilla (under the arm). In the simple or total mastectomy, the entire breast is removed. In limited procedures such as the "lumpectomy," or segmental mastectomy, the tumor plus a varying amount of surrounding tissue is removed.

Proponents of the more radical procedures think that they are necessary to eliminate all the cancerous tissue and prevent recurrence of the disease. The lymph nodes are removed because cancer is thought to spread first to the nodes and from there to distant sites in the body.

Proponents of the less extensive procedures think that the more radical procedures do not necessarily increase survival. They question the soundness of routine removal of unaffected lymph nodes since the nodes produce lymphocytes needed for cellular immunity, which is thought to be one of the body's major defenses against cancer. The radical procedures are also more traumatic both physically and psychologically.

FIGURE 25. Xeroradiogram showing carcinoma of the breast with calcifications (dark spots) indicative of this disease. [Source: Philip Strax, Guttman Institute, New York City]

Many investigators and clinicians, such as Bernard Fisher of the University of Pittsburgh School of Medicine, Pennsylvania, think that the current data are not adequate to resolve the controversy, which continues unabated. According to Fisher, since the data do not justify the conclusion that any of the procedures is any better or worse than any other, a clinical comparison of them is needed. Such a prospective, randomized clinical trial is now being conducted by the National Surgical Adjuvant Breast Project (NSABP) of which Fisher is chairman.

The study, which involves the cooperation of 35 medical institutions in the United States, includes about 1700 women who were operated on for breast cancer between September 1971 and August 1974. Those without node involvement, as determined by clinical examination, were randomly divided among three therapeutic modes: radical mastectomy, total mastectomy, or total mastectomy plus radiation of the nodes. According to Fisher, the preliminary results (as of September 1974) indicate no significant differences in the rates of cancer recurrence in the three groups of women.

Those with node involvement had either a radical mastectomy or a total mastectomy plus radiation to kill cancer cells in their lymph nodes. Again, no differences were observed between the two groups. If the results of this study hold up (survival for 5 years is the usual criterion for assessing cancer therapies), the next step may be a determination of the effectiveness of the segmental mastectomy.

Surgery and radiation have probably reached the limits of their effectiveness. Paul Carbone of NCI points out that approximately 30 percent of breast cancer patients are alive and free of disease 10 years after diagnosis—and this figure has remained constant for 35 years. These treatments can eradicate localized tumors but they cannot eliminate tumor cells or microscopic tumors harbored in other parts of the body. Only systemic treatments can reach these incipient tumors.

The most common systemic treatments now used for breast cancer are hormonal. They are employed only for recurrent or advanced inoperable disease. Some breast tumors depend on hormones, such as estrogen, for growth and maintenance. Removing the source of the hormone (the ovaries before menopause or the adrenals after it) or preventing its action by the use of androgens (male sex hormones) can slow tumor growth or even cause the tumor to regress. Since less than half of breast tumors respond to such therapy, the problem is determining which ones are responsive so that the other women can be spared unnecessary surgery.

An in vitro test currently undergoing clinical study may enable physicians to do just that. Elwood Jensen and his colleagues at the University of Chicago Medical School, Illinois, developed the test, which is based on the presence or absence of estrogen receptors in tumor cells. Estrogens, like other steroid hormones, must bind to these receptors before they can exert their effects on the cells. If the tumors lack receptors, they cannot respond to the hormones.

Jensen and his colleagues measured the estrogen-binding capacity of tumor samples taken during surgery or for biopsy. They found that in 26 of 36 patients whose cancer contained receptors, the tumor regressed in response to endocrine therapy. Of 43 patients whose tumors did not bind estrogens, only 1 responded. Thus, most patients with receptor-containing cancers benefit from hormone therapy, but there is little chance of benefit if the tumor cells lack receptors.

Chemotherapy is a systemic therapy that, until recently, was used only as a last resort for treating the most advanced cases of breast cancer. The current trend is for chemotherapy to be used as an adjunct to the primary treatment even though the patient may be clinically free of disease. The goal is the elimination of microscopic disseminated tumors that are not yet clinically apparent. In addition, clinicians are turning to drug combinations that are more effective than the agents administered separately.

In a preliminary study, George Cannellos and his colleagues at NCI found that a combination of four drugs—methotrexate, 5-fluorouracil, cyclophosphamide, and prednisone—caused regression of the tumors of 23 of 33 patients with advanced metastatic breast cancer. Seven patients had complete remissions. The median survival time of those who responded to the drug combination was at least double that of the nonresponders. In a more extensive collaborative study conducted by the Eastern Cooperative Oncology Group, consisting of 39 medical institutions in the eastern United States, the effectiveness of a single agent, L-phenylalanine mustard (L-PAM), was compared with that of a combination of three drugs. The combination produced both a greater response rate and a longer duration of response than did the single agent.

The NSABP is now coordinating clinical trials of L-PAM as an adjuvant to surgical treatment of breast cancer. Fisher said that the drug appears to prolong significantly the survival of patients with nodal involvement. The increased survival was particularly striking for younger patients who had not yet gone through menopause, but less significant for patients above the age of 49. As a result of this study, Fisher now routinely prescribes L-PAM for all younger patients whose cancer has spread to the lymph nodes. Studies of adjuvant chemotherapy with drug combinations are also planned.

Adjuvant chemotherapy, which may have hazardous side effects, may not be necessary for all patients. Carbone noted that patients whose breast cancer has not yet spread to the lymph nodes already have a good prognosis. In fact, the extent of nodal involvement is currently the best prognostic indicator, and this must be determined by examination of nodes removed during surgery because some of the involved nodes are not clinically detectable. This is another reason for performing the more extensive surgical procedures, which enable evaluation of the condition of the lymph nodes.

Other prognostic indicators, not requiring surgery, may eventually be available, however. Douglas Tormey and his associates at NCI found that more than 96 percent of patients with metastatic breast cancer have one or more of three biochemical markers—carcinoembryonic antigen, methylated guanosine, or human chorionic gonadotropin—in their blood or urine. Markers such as these may permit the identification of patients with a high risk of cancer recurrence without surgical removal of lymph nodes. Ultimately, Carbone says, clinicians hope to use a battery of diagnostic and prognostic tests to design the best treatment for each patient.

16
Leukemia

Much Is Known but the Picture Is Still Confused

If any type of human cancer is caused by a virus, it is probably leukemia. The virus may not be an infectious virus in the same sense as are those that cause polio and measles, but strong evidence is accumulating that some form of virus is involved in the etiology of leukemia. There is, however, a welter of evidence indicating that many other factors, including environmental influences and genetic predisposition, are also involved. The scenario presented by this evidence is complex, confusing, even contradictory, but this may be simply a reflection of the fact that more is known about leukemia than about any other type of cancer. The problems encountered in understanding and treating leukemia typify those found in other types of cancer and are illustrative of the general directions in which cancer research is headed.

Leukemia, cancer of the blood, is characterized by the uncontrolled proliferation and accumulation of leukocytes (white blood cells). Just as there are many different types of leukocytes, there are many different types of leukemia, but the four most important forms are derived from only two types of cells.

Acute and chronic lymphocytic leukemias (also known as lymphoblastic leukemias) are malignancies of lymphocytes, cells produced in the lymphoid organs (the spleen, lymph nodes, and thymus) and in the bone marrow. Lymphocytes can be divided into two morphologically indistinguishable subgroups, depending on their function. One subgroup, called thymus dependent or T cells, is involved in the phenomenon known as cellular immunity, the process by which the body distinguishes between self and nonself. The second subgroup, thymus independent or B cells, controls the production of circulating antibodies, substances that attack infectious microorganisms. Recent research by Jun Minowada and his associates at Roswell Park Memorial Institute, Buffalo, New York, and by others suggests that acute lymphocytic leukemia is a disorder of T cells, while chronic lymphocytic leukemia is a disorder of B cells.

Acute and chronic myelocytic leukemias (also known as granulocytic or myelogenous leukemias) are disorders of granulocytes. Granulocytes, produced by bone marrow, engulf and digest bacteria and other small particles. There is as yet no evidence to support a biochemical distinction between the acute and chronic forms of myelocytic leukemia.

Acute leukemias generally appear suddenly, with symptoms like those of a cold, and progress rapidly. The lymph nodes, spleen, and liver may become infiltrated with leukocytes and enlarged; there is often bone pain, paleness, a tendency to bleed easily, and a high susceptibility to infections. The most common causes of death, which occurs at a median of 3 months without treatment, are hemorrhaging and uncontrolled infections. The chronic leukemias begin much more slowly; many cases are discovered during routine blood examinations, and several years may pass before significant symptoms appear. The symptoms are similar to those of the acute leukemias, but the life expectancy without treatment is about 3 years after onset.

Acute lymphocytic leukemia is the most common cancer of childhood (about 3000 cases per year), but it is more common in adults. Acute myelocytic leukemia occurs much less frequently in children, and the chronic forms occur almost exclusively in adults. Leukemias strike about 19,000 individuals in the United States each year and take the lives of approximately 14,000.

For many years, it was assumed that the symptoms of leukemia arose because leukemic leukocytes proliferated much more rapidly than healthy ones. In 1953, however, the Italian investigators G. Astaldi and C. Mauri demonstrated that leukemic cells actually proliferate more slowly than their healthy counterparts (although there are occasional periods of rapid growth). Subsequent work by many investigators has shown that the primary lesion in leukemia is a block in the differentiation of leukocytes. Most leukemic cells never mature into functional entities. Not only is the body thus deprived of vital components of its immune system, but also the cells accumulate in the blood and in certain organs, forcing out healthy cells and interfering with organ function.

The proximate cause of the block in maturation is still unknown, but many scientists think it results from the loss of a specific factor necessary for maturation. In 1966, Leo Sachs of the Weizmann Institute in Rehovot, Israel, developed a system for growing leukemic cells in culture. Using this system, he and Michael Perrin, now at the National Cancer Institute (NCI) in Bethesda, Maryland, demonstrated that cultured leukocytes from patients with acute myelocytic leukemia could apparently be induced to mature in the presence of a particular glycoprotein from blood serum. This substance is called colony-stimulating factor (CSF) because the mature cells form colonies in the culture.

CSF is present in the blood of leukemia patients, but it is not yet clear whether its concentration is lower in these patients than in healthy individuals or whether a membrane defect prevents CSF from exerting its normal control over differentiation. The former possibility is supported somewhat by observations indicating that systemic factors are important. Alvin M. Mauer of the University of Cincinnati, Ohio, for example, has shown that the proliferative activity of leukemic cells is the same at different bone marrow sites, indicating that some substance in the blood regulates the leukemic process.

But there is no firm evidence, argue some scientists, such as Fred Stohlman of St. Elizabeth's Hospital, Boston, Massachusetts, that the CSF-induced changes are a functional maturation, and a great deal more work will be necessary before any conclusions can be drawn about the role of CSF. In any case, work on CSF is proceeding very slowly: There is no rapid assay for CSF, and this makes its isolation very tedious. Sachs and others have argued that it may be very useful in treating human leukemia, but a demonstration of this possibility is probably far in the future.

If the proximate cause of blocked maturation is a mystery, so too is the ultimate cause. But perhaps the greatest excitement in leukemia research today surrounds the possibility that human leukemia may be caused by a virus. It has long been recognized that leukemia (and other cancers arising in mesenchymal cells) can be triggered in several species of animals—rodents, cats, cows, birds, and subhuman primates—by agents known as type C RNA tumor viruses or oncornaviruses. Many virologists think that human leukemias should not differ grossly from these animal leukemias.

Oncornaviruses replicate in infected cells through the mediation of an enzyme known as RNA-directed DNA polymerase or reverse transcriptase. Reverse transcriptase directs the production of a DNA copy of the virus's RNA genome. This copy, called the provirus, then serves as a template for production by the host cell of more RNA viruses. More important, the provirus can be inserted into the DNA genome of the host cell—where, if the virus contains oncogenic (tumor-initiating) information, it can assume control of the host cell's proliferation and transform it into a malignant cell. To date, all oncogenic RNA viruses have been shown to contain a reverse transcriptase and virtually all RNA viruses that contain a reverse transcriptase have been shown to be oncogenic. But despite a great deal of effort by many investigators and with only one possible exception, a reverse transcriptase has never been found in any nonmalignant cell not infected by an oncornavirus.

In 1970, Robert C. Gallo and his associates at NCI demonstrated that granulocytes from humans with acute myelocytic leukemia contain a reverse transcriptase analogous to those found in oncornaviruses. Subsequently, Sol Spiegelman and his associates at the Institute for Cancer Research at Columbia University, New York City, and Gallo have independently shown that the reverse transcriptase is found in a cytoplasmic particle which has the same density as oncornaviruses and which also contains RNA of a size characteristic of oncornaviruses. Both groups have shown by molecular hybridization experiments that DNA produced by the RNA–reverse transcriptase complex contains base sequences homologous to those of mouse leukemia and sarcoma viruses but does not contain sequences homologous to those of avian oncornaviruses or of a mouse type B RNA virus (mouse mammary tumor virus). Gallo and David Gillespie of Litton Bionetics, Bethesda, Maryland, have also shown that this DNA contains even more sequences homologous to those in simian sarcoma virus, an oncornavirus that produces a leukemialike disease in primates.

Gallo and his associates have purified the reverse transcriptase from leukemic granulocytes and have shown that it accepts the same types of nucleic acid templates as do the enzymes from animal oncornaviruses. And finally, he and George J. Todaro of NCI have shown that the purified enzyme is immunologically very closely related to the reverse transcriptases from simian sarcoma virus and from gibbon ape leukemia virus, less closely related to those from mouse and cat oncornaviruses, and unrelated to that from a chicken oncornavirus. Since many scientists now accept the postulate that reverse transcriptase is unequivocally associated with cell transformation by RNA viruses, the presence in leukemic human cells of a reverse transcriptase closely related to those of viruses that cause leukemia in other primates is highly suggestive of the possibility that human leukemia is caused by an RNA virus.

Spiegelman, meanwhile, has demonstrated that DNA produced by the RNA–reverse transcriptase complex from human granulocytes contains sequences that will not hybridize with DNA from healthy tissues (muscle, for example) from the same patient. This finding suggests that extra—presumably oncogenic—genetic information has been added to the genome of bone marrow cells sometime after birth. This hypothesis is supported by experiments with identical human twins, one of whom has leukemia. By hybridization experiments, Spiegelman has shown for two sets of twins that the leukocyte genome of the leukemic twin contains DNA sequences not present in leukocytes of the healthy twin, again suggesting that oncogenic information has been added after birth.

Gallo's and Spiegelman's results are by far the strongest evidence supporting viral involvement in leukemia, but a recent observation by E. Donnall Thomas of the University of Washington School of Medicine, Seattle, adds further support. Thomas has been treating terminal myelocytic leukemia patients by destroying their bone marrow with drugs or radiation and transplanting healthy bone marrow from a donor. In this manner, all the leukemic cells can be killed and the healthy grafted cells can take their place; The primary problems with this approach are obtaining bone marrow that will not be rejected and preventing infections during the period before the grafted cells begin functioning. Most investigators have been largely unsuccessful in their attempts at grafting bone marrow.

By improving the immunological match between the patient and the donor, Thomas has had better success with the grafts than most investigators have, but he has recently observed two interesting cases in which the patient had a relapse of leukemia. Subsequent examination of chromosomes from the leukemic cells indicated that they were from the male donor rather than from the female patient, indicating that the patient harbored some agent—possibly viral—capable of transforming the transplanted cells.

The ultimate proof of the viral hypothesis would be the isolation of a leukemia virus from humans, and that possibility is beginning to appear more likely. For example, Boris Lapin of the Institute of Pathology and Therapy at Sukhumia in the U.S.S.R. has claimed that he and his associates have succeeded in inducing leukemia in primates by inoculating them with blood from human leukemia patients and have isolated what they believe to be a human type C RNA leukemia virus. U.S. scientists have not been able to duplicate Lapin's experiments and have obtained only equivocal results with materials provided by him. However, NCI has received one of Lapin's leukemic baboons, and preliminary experiments with this animal have been described by NCI officials as promising. And early in 1975, Gallo and Robert E. Gallagher of NCI announced that they have isolated a type C RNA virus from a patient with acute myelocytic leukemia. They believe it to be a human leukemia virus.

Despite all the evidence implicating viruses in human leukemia, it is clear that a number of other factors are also involved. The most important of these are chromosomal aberrations. Evidence is increasing that environmentally induced and genetically determined chromosome breakage and genetically determined chromosome breakage and rearrangement increase the incidence of leukemia.

A well-established environmental cause of leukemia is radiation, as is deduced from the much higher incidence among radiologists (before protective precautions began to be taken routinely) and among survivors of the nuclear blasts that ended World War II. Radiation increases the incidence of all types of leukemia except chronic lymphocytic leukemia. The principal leukemogenic effect of irradiation is believed to be breakage of chromosomes in bone marrow cells (but radiation is also known to activate latent viruses). Similarly, benzene, the only chemical thought to be leukemogenic, also induces breakage in bone marrow chromosomes. But genetic factors apparently play a more important role in leukemogenesis, even when radiation is present. Studies of the Hiroshima and Nagasaki survivors by the Atomic Bomb Casualty Commission indicate that only 1 of every 100 individuals exposed to the highest levels of radiation contracted leukemia.

In 1960, Peter Nowell and David Hungerford of the University of Pennsylvania, Philadelphia, observed that more than 90 percent of patients with chronic myelocytic leukemia (and a small fraction of patients with the acute form) have a specific chromosomal abnormality: The long arm of chromosome number 22 from their granulocytes—now known as the Philadelphia chromosome—is shorter than its counterpart in cells from healthy tissues. Last year, Janet D. Rowley of the University of Chicago, Illinois, found that these patients have additional DNA in their chromosome number 9 and that the mass of the added material is about equal to that missing from chromosome number 22. It thus seems likely that translocation of genetic information from chromosome number 22 to chromosome number 9 may cause or increase the incidence of leukemia.

Certain other types of genetic disorders also predispose to a greater incidence of leukemia. For example, children with Down's syndrome (mongolism), a genetic defect characterized by mental retardation and certain other abnormalities, have a 15-fold higher incidence of acute leukemia than have normal children. The specific genetic lesion in Down's syndrome, is the presence of an extra chromosome number 21. Similarly, about 10 percent of children with Fanconi's aplastic anemia, a genetic defect in which all blood components show a reduced proliferation, develop acute monomyelocytic leukemia, a rare form that accounts for less than 4 percent of all leukemias.

There are, according to Robert Miller of NCI, several other genetic defects that are associated with a high incidence of leukemia. The common feature that links these defects, he says, is chromosomal fragility; that is, each of the disorders makes the afflicted individual's chromosomes more susceptible to breakage and rearrangement. It may be, Miller says, that breakage makes cells more susceptible to viral infection or to expression of latent viruses, but it is also possible that rearrangement and defective repair of DNA may lead to inappropriate expression of genes, a condition that is also thought to be oncogenic in some instances.

There is some evidence that induction of leukemia may be associated with breakage at specific chromosomes sites. Fred Hecht of the University of Oregon Medical School, Portland, has presented evidence that in one genetic disorder, ataxia telangiectasia (characterized by failure of muscular coordination, pulmonary disease, and abnormal eye movements), the occurrence of preleukemic lymphocyte proliferation in several patients and of chronic lymphocytic leukemia in at least one patient is associated with breakage of chromosome number 14. This finding is consistent, Hecht says, with the observation by other investigators that breakages in chromosome number 14 are found in patients with Burkitt's lymphoma, a leukemialike tumor of the lymph gland.

Genetic factors not associated with fragility are also linked to leukemia. Among white children, for example, there is a marked peak in mortality from acute lymphocytic leukemia at the age of 4 years. This peak occurs at the age of 1 in children with Down's syndrome, and does not occur at all in black children. An identical twin has a much greater risk of contracting leukemia if his twin has already done so. For the second twin, this risk declines from about 100 percent if the first contracted leukemia before age 1 to about 20 percent if he contracted it at age 6. It is thus clear that a wide variety of effects are implicated in the induction of leukemia. There may eventually be some hypothesis that will reconcile all the seemingly contradictory data, but for now the etiology of leukemia remains an enigma.

The accumulation of knowledge about leukemia has contributed to the success of therapy for leukemia patients. Perhaps the most important of these contributions was obtained from a knowledge of the kinetics of leukemic cell proliferation, which has allowed chemotherapists to design much more effective drug schedules. Knowledge of some of the biochemical pathways of leukemic cells has provided guidance in the use of antimetabolites, drugs that interfere with the cell's metabolism. And the discovery of reverse transcriptase in leukemic cells has sparked a great deal of research for inhibitors of the enzyme and of viral replication. Nevertheless, most of the therapeutic advances in leukemia have resulted from the same sort of sophisticated trial-and-error techniques necessary in other types of cancer. The task of devising therapies has been made all the harder by the greatly different susceptibilities of the various types of leukemia and by age-dependent differences within any one type.

The greatest success in leukemia therapy has been achieved in treating children with acute lymphocytic leukemia. Twenty years ago, the median survival for children with this disease was about 3 months, and even as recently as about 12 years ago, chemotherapy was expected to be no more than palliative. Today, the median survival is 5 years, and many afflicted children have been alive for 10 years or longer.

It is difficult to identify individuals who have made the greatest contributions to this achievement because the effort has been largely a group one. Leukemia patients are encountered so infrequently that significant results from clinical studies can be obtained only by pooling results from patients treated at many institutions. Changes or improvements in drug regimens are thus frequently a matter of group consensus rather than individual choice.

Leukemia chemotherapy began in 1947 when the late Sidney Farber of the Children's Cancer Research Foundation in Boston, Massachusetts, started obtaining brief remissions with the antimetabolites aminopterin and methotrexate. Many of the concepts now used in leukemia therapy were later developed at NCI by Emil J. Freireich, who is now at the M. D. Anderson Hospital and Tumor Institute, Houston, Texas. Some of the best results are now being obtained by Donald Pinkel and Joseph Simone at St. Jude Children's Research Hospital in Memphis, Tennessee, one of the few institutions with enough patients to conduct clinical trials independently.

Pinkel and Simone's regimen, typical of those used at other institutions, includes induction of a remission with vincristine and steroid hormones, x-irradiation to destroy leukemic lymphocytes harbored in the central nervous system, and a 3-year course of chemotherapy consisting of daily doses of 6-mercaptopurine and weekly doses of methotrexate (Table 6). An initial remission is obtained in about 90 percent of children under the age of 10. In their first series of studies, which lasted from 1962 to 1965, Pinkel and Simone used what is now recognized to be an insufficient dose of radiation, but 7 of 41 children in those studies are still alive. With a larger radiation dose in subsequent studies, 19 of 38 children

TABLE 6

The Evolution of Leukemia Therapy at St. Jude Children's Research Hospital in Memphis
[Source: Joseph V. Simone]

Study and years	Remission induction	Intensive chemotherapy phase	Preventive CNS therapy	Continuation chemotherapy
I 1962	Pred + VCR	None	500 rads craniospinal	6-MP P.O. daily VCR i.v. weekly Cyclo i.v. weekly
II 1963	Pred + VCR	None	500 rads craniospinal	6-MP P.O. daily or MTX i.m. weekly VCR i.v. every 2 wk Cyclo i.v. every 2 wk
III 1964–1965	Pred + VCR	6-MP i.v. daily × 3 MTX i.v. daily × 3 Cyclo i.v. X 1	1200 rads craniospinal	6-MP P.O. daily MTX, Cyclo, and VCR i.v. weekly
IV 1965–1967	Pred + VCR	As in III	None	Full or half dosage 6-MP P.O. daily MTX, Cyclo, and VCR i.v. weekly

V 1967–1968	Pred + VCR	As in III	2400 rads cranial + i.t. MTX	6-MP P.O. daily MTX i.v. weekly Cyclo i.v. weekly Pred + VCR, 2-wk course every 10 wk
VI 1968–1970	Pred + VCR + Dauno	As in III or none	2400 rads craniospinal or none	6-MP P.O. daily MTX P.O. weekly Cyclo P.O. weekly Pred + VCR, 2-wk course every 12 wk
VII 1970–1971	Pred + VCR	None	2400 rads cranial + i.t. MTX or 2400 rads craniospinal	6-MP P.O. daily MTX P.O. weekly Cyclo P.O. weekly Pred + VCR, 2-wk course every 12 wk
VIII 1972–	Pred + VCR + Asp	None	2400 rads cranial + i.t. MTX	MTX i.v. weekly 6-MP P.O. daily Cyclo i.v. weekly + Ara-C i.v. weekly

Pred = prednisone;   VCR = vincristine;   6-MP = 6-mercaptopurine;   Ara-C = cytosine   arabinoside;   Cyclo = cyclophosphamide;
MTX = methotrexate; Dauno = daunorubicin; Asp = L-asparaginase. Results of the studies are presented in the text.

are still alive after six or more years. And only 1 of 40 children in current studies has had a relapse after $2\frac{1}{2}$ years. Similar results have been obtained by the Acute Leukemia Group B, a consortium of 56 clinical groups in the northeastern United States, whose chairman is James F. Holland of the Mt. Sinai School of Medicine, New York City.

A major contribution to the success of these antileukemic regimens has been the development of supportive therapy to counteract the side effects of leukemia. The most important of these are hemorrhaging, caused by loss of platelets from the blood, and a high susceptibility to infectious diseases, resulting from suppression of the immune system by both the leukemia and the chemotherapeutic agents.

The hemorrhaging can be controlled by transfusing the patient with platelets, but obtaining platelets was once a major problem. In the late 1950's however, Isaac Djerassi, now at the Mercy Catholic Medical Center, Darby, Pennsylvania, and Edmund Klein, now at Roswell Park Memorial Institute, and, independently, Freireich developed methods for removing platelets from blood and returning the red blood cells to the donor. With this technique, one donor can now provide a continuing supply of platelets for a leukemia victim. More recently, Freireich and Djerassi have independently developed a similar plasmapheresis technique for collecting functional granulocytes from patients with chronic myelocytic leukemia. These patients produce much greater quantities of granulocytes than do healthy persons, and as many as ten leukemia patients can be helped by one donor. Transfused into compatible patients with acute lymphocytic leukemia, these granulocytes help fight off infections while the patient's own immune system is recovering.

A remission of acute lymphocytic leukemia for five or more years is frequently considered to be a cure—or the next best thing to one. Some recent evidence, however, suggests that the potential for a relapse still exists within these patients. By molecular hybridization experiments with the probe described previously, Spiegelman has shown that lymphocytes from many of these long-term survivors still contain presumably oncogenic DNA sequences not found in corresponding cells from healthy individuals. This finding, he says, indicates that the therapeutic regimen has removed the symptoms of the malignancy but not the underlying cause, so that the symptoms may recur at a later date.

The success in treating acute lymphocytic leukemia in children is not even approached in adults with the same disease. The median survival of the patient varies inversely with his age at onset of the disease: The older the patient, the less susceptible he is to therapy. Drugs such as vincristine and prednisone, which produce a high rate of remissions in young children, are only minimally effective in adults. Treatment with newer drugs, such as adriamycin and arabinosylcytosine, has been somewhat successful, but the median survival for adults is still less than 1 year.

The present status of therapy for acute myelocytic leukemia, according to Myron Karon of the Los Angeles Children's Hospital, California, is similar to that for acute lymphocytic leukemia about 4 years ago. An initial remission can now be obtained in about 80 percent of patients with acute myelocytic leukemia, compared to only 30 percent a few years ago. The median survival, similarly, has been extended from 1 month to about 18 months.

Because acute myelocytic leukemia is more resistant to therapy than is acute lymphocytic leukemia, one approach to its control, pioneered by Freireich, involves an intensified course of chemotherapy—higher doses given more frequently. But this regimen greatly depresses the patient's immune system, making him much more susceptible to infections. Freireich therefore isolates the patients in laminar air-flow bedrooms in a sterile environment (Figure 27). Of 20 patients treated in this fashion, 15 are still in remission with a median disease-free period of about 2 years. Some scientists, however, are skeptical as to whether the sterile environment is a necessary facet of the protocol and Freireich is beginning a clinical study to determine whether it is.

The outlook for both chronic lymphocytic leukemia and chronic myelocytic leukemia is much less promising, according to Paul Carbone of NCI. The median survival in both types is less than 3 years and has not been improved by any form of therapy, probably because the chronic types have generally received only minimal treatment. There is some prospect for improvement, however, because clinicians are beginning to treat the chronic diseases much more aggressively. For instance, Bayerd Clarkson of Memorial Sloan-Kettering Cancer Center, New York City, has found that an aggressive protocol that includes removal of the spleen, radiation, and intensive chemotherapy produces a high rate of remissions

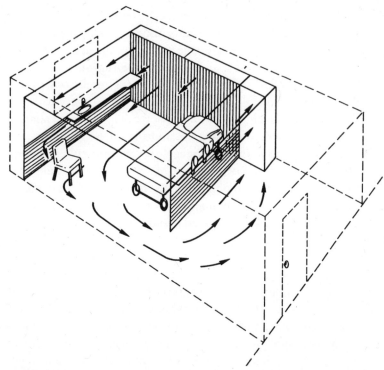

FIGURE 27. One type of laminar air flow bedroom. The unit at the head of the bed cleans and circulates air in a hospital room so that airborne infectious agents are kept away from the patient. [Source: National Cancer Institute]

in adults with chronic myelocytic leukemia. This approach seems particularly promising because in 4 of 25 patients, it had led to the disappearance of the Philadelphia chromosome, the genetic marker associated with the disease, but the protocol has been in use for too short a time for a full assessment.

Therapy of leukemia thus encompasses the full range of possibilities, from a high percentage of potential cures in children with acute lymphocytic leukemia to almost none in adults with chronic lymphocytic leukemia. It is clear, however, that progress is being made in treatment of each type of the disease and especially in obtaining a greater knowledge of its molecular biology. The knowledge of leukemia that is being rapidly obtained opens many new areas of potential therapy and even prevention. And in the end, that is what cancer research is all about.

Appendix

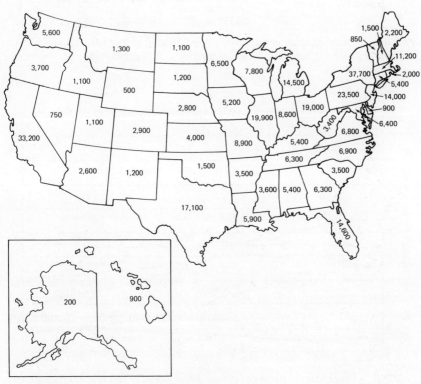

FIGURE 28. Geographical distribution of estimated U.S. cancer deaths, 1974. The estimated total number of deaths is 355,000. [Source: American Cancer Society]

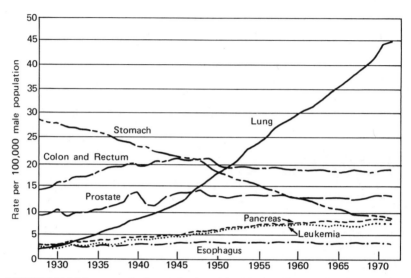

FIGURE 29. Male cancer death rates by site, United States, 1930–1969. The rates are for the male population standardized for age on the 1940 U.S. population. [Source: American Cancer Society]

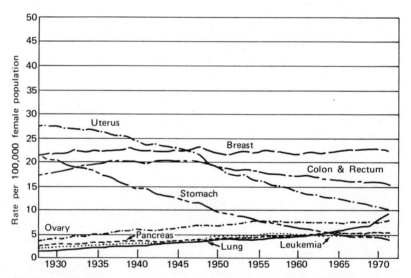

FIGURE 30. Female cancer death rates by site, United States, 1930–1969. The rates are for the female population standardized for age on the 1940 U.S. population. [Source: American Cancer Society]

TABLE 7

Relation of Cancer to Other Leading Causes of Death in the United States, 1969
[Source: American Cancer Society]

Rank	Cause of death	Number of deaths	Death rate per 100,000 population	Percent of total deaths
	ALL CAUSES	1,921,990	951.9	100.0
1	Diseases of heart	738,945	359.9	38.4
2	Cancer	323,092	160.0	16.8
3	Stroke (cerebrovascular disease)	207,179	102.6	10.8
4	Accidents	116,385	57.6	6.1
	Motor vehicle accidents	55,791	27.6	2.9
	All other accidents	60,594	30.0	3.2
5	Influenza and pneumonia	68,365	33.9	3.6
6	Certain diseases of early infancy	43,171	21.4	2.2
7	Diabetes mellitus	38,541	19.1	2.0
8	Arteriosclerosis	33,063	16.4	1.7
9	Cirrhosis of liver	29,866	14.8	1.6
10	Emphysema	22,939	11.4	1.2
11	Suicide	22,364	11.1	1.2
12	Congenital anomalies	17,008	8.4	0.9
13	Homicide	15,477	7.7	0.8
14	Nephritis and nephrosis	9416	4.7	0.5
15	Infections of kidney	8750	4.3	0.5
16	All others	227,428	61.0	11.8

TABLE 8

Estimated Cancer Deaths and New Cases by Sex and Site, 1973*

[Source: American Cancer Society]

Site	Estimated deaths			Estimated new cases		
	Total	Male	Female	Total	Male	Female
All sites	350,000	190,000	160,000	665,000	344,000	321,000
Buccal cavity and pharynx (oral)	7,600	5,550	2,050	15,400	10,500	4,900
Lip	175	150	25	1,900	1,700	200
Tongue	1,750	1,300	450	2,800	1,900	900
Salivary gland	650	400	250			
Floor of mouth	525	400	125	6000	3600	2,400
Other and unspecified mouth	1,100	700	400			
Pharynx	3,400	2,600	800	4,700	3,300	1,400
Digestive organs	97,300	51,600	45,700	132,600	69,000	63,600
Esophagus	6,400	4,700	1,700	6,800	5,100	1,700
Stomach	14,700	8,700	6,000	16,400	9,700	6,700
Small intestine	750	400	350	1,200	700	500
Large intestine (Colon–	37,000	17,100	19,900	57,000	26,000	31,000
Rectum)	10,400	5,800	4,600	22,000	12,000	10,000
Liver (specified as primary)	7,200	3,200	4,000	7,300	3,300	4,000
Pancreas	19,200	10,900	8,300	19,400	11,000	8,400
Other and unspecified digestive	1,650	800	850	2,500	1,200	1,300
Respiratory system	76,250	61,300	14,950	88,600	71,500	17,100
Larynx	3,050	2,700	350	6,900	6,000	900
Lung	72,000	57,900	14,100	79,000	64,000	15,000
Other and unspecified respiratory	1,200	700	500	2,700	1,500	1,200
Bone, tissue, and skin	8,750	5,100	3,650	127,700	82,000	45,700
Bone	1,900	1,100	800	1,900	1,000	900
Connective tissue	1,650	900	750	5,800	3,000	2,800
Skin	5,200	3,100	2,100	120,000	78,000	42,000

Breast	*32,650*	*250*	*32,400*	*73,600*	*600*	*73,000*
Genital organs	42,000	18,800	23,200	102,500	40,400	62,100
Cervix uteri ⎫ *(uterus)*	*8,700*	*—*	*8,700*	*46,000*	*—*	*46,000*
Corpus uteri ⎭	3,100	—	3,100			
Ovary	10,500	—	10,500	14,000	—	14,000
Other female genital	900	—	900	2,100	—	2,100
Prostate	17,800	17,800	—	38,000	38,000	—
Other male genital	1,000	1,000	—	2,400	2,400	—
Urinary organs	16,000	10,500	5,500	32,200	22,000	10,200
Bladder	9,200	6,300	2,900	20,800	15,000	5,800
Kidney and other urinary	6,800	4,200	2,600	11,400	7,000	4,400
Eye	350	150	200	600	300	300
Brain and central nervous system	8,000	4,700	3,300	11,700	6,400	5,300
Endocrine glands	1,650	650	1000	3,600	1,100	2,500
Thyroid	1,150	350	800	2,900	700	2,200
Other endocrine	500	300	200	700	400	300
Leukemia	15,300	8,600	6,700	19,000	11,000	8,000
Lymphomas	20,300	11,100	9,200	25,500	14,200	11,300
Lymphosarcoma and reticulosarcoma	7,700	4,100	3,600	10,600	6,000	4,600
Hodgkin's disease	3,700	2,200	1,500	4,800	2,700	2,100
Multiple myeloma	4,600	2,400	2,200	10,100	5,500	4,600
Other lymphomas	4,300	2,400	1,900			
All other and unspecified sites	23,850	11,700	12,150	32,000	15,000	17,000

*The figures do not include carcinoma-in-situ of the uterus (about 40,000 cases per year) and superficial skin cancer (between 300,000 and 600,000 cases per year). The estimates are not definitive. The six major sites are in italics.

TABLE 9

Percentage of Patients with Various Types of Cancer Who Survive for 3 or 5 Years*

[Source: National Cancer Institute]

Primary site	Percent of all cancers			3-Year relative survival rate			5-Year relative survival rate		
	Total	Male	Female	Total	Male	Female	Total	Male	Female
Total all sites	100.0	100.0	100.0	45	37	53	40	31	47
Lip	1.2	2.2	0.2	91	91	95	87	87	89
Tongue	1.2	1.7	0.6	39	35	52	32	27	47
Salivary gland	1.2	1.0	1.3	89	83	94	88	81	93
Floor of mouth	0.7	1.0	0.3	50	47	60	43	40	52
Other mouth	0.8	1.1	0.5	52	50	56	45	41	52
Mesopharynx	0.7	1.0	0.3	37	34	44	29	27	37
Nasopharynx	0.3	0.4	0.2	36	34	42	28	26	34
Hypopharynx	0.4	0.7	0.1	23	22	25	17	16	23
Esophagus	1.5	2.3	0.7	6	5	9	3	2	7
Stomach	4.5	5.7	3.4	15	15	16	12	11	14
Ascending colon, caecum, appendix	2.7	2.1	3.3	51	48	53	48	43	51
Transverse colon	1.3	1.2	1.5	46	44	47	41	38	43
Descending colon	0.7	0.6	0.8	53	53	54	46	44	47
Sigmoid colon	3.3	3.2	3.5	53	52	54	47	45	48
Rectum	5.2	5.7	4.8	47	45	49	40	38	41
Liver	0.4	0.5	0.3	3	2	5	3	1	6
Gallbladder and ducts	1.1	0.8	1.4	10	9	10	7	7	8
Pancreas	2.4	2.8	2.0	2	2	2	1	1	2
Nose, nasal cavities, middle ear	0.4	0.5	0.3	46	44	49	40	39	41
Larynx	2.0	3.6	0.4	61	61	60	55	56	53
Lung and bronchus	10.3	17.2	3.1	11	10	14	8	8	11
Female breast	11.8	—	23.8	—	—	72	—	—	52
Cervix uteri	4.8	—	9.8	—	—	65	—	—	60

Corpus uteri	3.5	—	7.0	—	—	—	75	—	72
Ovary	2.4	—	4.8	—	—	—	36	—	32
Vulva	0.4	—	0.9	—	—	—	66	—	62
Vagina	0.2	—	0.3	—	—	—	44	—	36
Prostate	6.3	12.4	—	—	63	—	—	51	—
Testis	0.5	0.9	—	—	66	—	—	65	—
Penis	0.2	0.3	—	—	73	—	—	69	—
Kidney	1.8	2.2	1.4	42	41	44	36	35	38
Bladder	4.6	6.7	2.5	60	60	59	56	56	56
Melanoma of skin	1.3	1.2	1.3	68	61	74	61	53	68
Eye	0.5	0.6	0.5	86	85	86	80	81	78
Brain and cranial meninges	2.6	2.7	2.5	31	28	35	28	24	33
Thyroid gland	1.3	0.7	1.9	84	77	86	82	75	85
Bone	0.5	0.5	0.4	40	36	44	35	32	38
Connective tissue	0.9	1.0	0.9	54	51	58	50	46	53
Reticulum cell sarcoma	0.5	0.6	0.5	20	21	20	16	17	15
Lymphosarcoma	0.9	1.0	0.8	40	40	39	29	30	28
Hodgkin's disease	1.1	1.3	0.9	50	46	55	39	36	44
Other forms of lymphoma	0.3	0.3	0.3	54	53	55	44	42	46
Multiple myeloma	0.8	0.9	0.8	17	17	16	9	9	9
Acute lymphocytic leukemia	0.5	0.6	0.4	5	5	5	2	2	3
Acute myelocytic leukemia	0.5	0.6	0.5	1	1	1	1	1	1
Monocytic leukemia	0.4	0.4	0.4	3	3	3	1	2	1
Acute leukemia (not otherwise specified)	0.4	0.4	0.3	4	3	5	2	1	2
Chronic lymphocytic leukemia	1.0	1.3	0.8	51	49	55	38	34	43
Chronic myelocytic leukemia	0.7	0.7	0.6	25	22	28	13	11	14
Other and unspecified sites	7.0	7.4	6.7	—	—	—	—	—	—

* The relative survival rate effectively eliminates the patients who die from causes other than cancer. Data is for cancers diagnosed from 1955 to 1964.

TABLE 10

Age-Adjusted Death Rates per 100,000 Population for Selected Cancer Sites for 39 Countries, 1966–1967

[Source: American Cancer Society]

Country	All sites Male	All sites Female	Oral Male	Oral Female	Colon and rectum Male	Colon and rectum Female	Lung Male	Lung Female
United States	150.6 (17)*	106.7 (19)	4.55 (8)	1.31 (13)	18.79 (12)	16.09 (11)	40.24 (10)	6.75 (12)
Australia	143.2 (21)	96.8 (29)	3.57 (14)	1.08 (17)	18.18 (14)	17.08 (9)	37.64 (12)	4.77 (24)
Austria	192.7 (3)	130.3 (4)	3.07 (16)	0.81 (24)	20.58 (7)	14.92 (12)	50.35 (6)	6.09 (14)
Belgium	182.9 (5)	120.3 (8)	2.38 (25)	0.58 (36)	20.99 (5)	18.14 (6)	50.09 (7)	4.36 (21)
Bulgaria	136.3 (25)	85.1 (32)	1.99 (29)	0.66 (32)	7.05 (28)	6.22 (29)	36.00 (16)	6.72 (13)
Canada	146.8 (19)	109.0 (16)	4.11 (10)	1.09 (16)	21.51 (3)	19.02 (4)	34.52 (18)	5.36 (19)
Chile	149.8 (18)	137.1 (1)	2.06 (28)	0.76 (28)	4.03 (35)	2.45 (37)	15.18 (29)	5.59 (17)
China	102.2 (35)	74.0 (34)	6.37 (3)	2.95 (3)	15.13 (18)	8.61 (25)	10.02 (33)	5.45 (18)
Columbia	38.2 (36)	99.4 (27)	2.16 (27)	1.75 (6)	3.58 (36)	3.77 (35)	7.26 (36)	3.57 (31)
Czechoslovakia	197.5 (2)	101.4 (24)	2.93 (18)	0.75 (30)	13.01 (2)	11.11 (20)	59.98 (4)	5.68 (16)
Denmark	158.2 (14)	132.6 (2)	1.83 (31)	0.89 (22)	22.96 (2)	19.30 (3)	37.34 (15)	7.36 (8)
Dominican Rep.	31.6 (39)	35.6 (39)	1.11 (38)	0.61 (35)	1.78 (38)	1.91 (38)	3.19 (37)	1.84 (38)
England & Wales	182.5 (6)	114.9 (11)	2.92 (21)	1.41 (11)	21.36 (4)	17.10 (8)	69.66 (2)	10.73 (3)
Finland	183.1 (4)	102.8 (22)	2.93 (19)	0.99 (13)	10.76 (24)	9.08 (24)	61.00 (3)	3.91 (30)
France	174.1 (8)	100.3 (25)	9.96 (2)	0.79 (25)	18.55 (13)	13.78 (14)	27.71 (23)	3.74 (32)
Germany (F.R.)	174.1 (9)	126.5 (5)	1.80 (32)	0.51 (37)	18.99 (10)	14.69 (13)	42.09 (9)	5.10 (22)
Greece	123.9 (29)	73.5 (35)	1.28 (37)	0.55 (38)	4.94 (33)	4.87 (33)	31.32 (20)	6.05 (15)
Hong Kong	170.4 (11)	102.1 (23)	19.77 (1)	7.63 (1)	15.14 (18)	8.61 25	84.16 (17)	18.28 (1)
Hungary	166.8 (12)	120.1 (9)	3.81 (12)	0.72 (31)	15.51 (17)	13.52 (15)	37.36 (14)	7.23 (9)
Iceland	132.8 (26)	131.1 (3)	2.41 (23)	2.66 (4)	11.75 (23)	9.91 (23)	15.25 (28)	8.63 (4)
Ireland	142.9 (22)	115.1 (10)	4.39 (9)	1.49 (10)	19.34 (9)	18.47 (5)	33.54 (19)	7.88 (5)
Israel	121.5 (30)	114.5 (12)	1.38 (35)	0.78 (26)	10.60 (25)	10.50 (22)	22.51 (26)	7.62 (7)
Italy	152.0 (15)	99.3 (28)	5.39 (6)	0.94 (2)	14.23 (19)	10.74 (21)	30.23 (21)	4.53 (25)
Japan	141.3 (24)	94.9 (30)	1.38 (36)	0.63 (33)	8.22 (26)	7.06 (26)	13.97 (31)	4.86 (22)
Mexico	53.3 (38)	71.9 (37)	1.48 (34)	0.62 (34)	2.76 (37)	3.39 (36)	7.30 (35)	4.07 (29)
Netherlands	175.5 (7)	120.7 (7)	1.52 (33)	0.75 (29)	17.47 (15)	16.60 (10)	53.63 (5)	3.42 (34)
New Zealand	146.2 (20)	109.5 (14)	2.39 (24)	1.15 (15)	20.39 (8)	19.77 (2)	37.72 (11)	5.35 (20)
Northern Ireland	151.3 (16)	107.0 (18)	3.80 (11)	1.97 (5)	20.91 (6)	17.78 (7)	43.29 (8)	7.14 (10)
Norway	124.7 (28)	100.1 (26)	2.21 (25)	1.63 (7)	13.47 (20)	12.02 (18)	14.93 (30)	2.97 (35)
Panama	81.6 (37)	67.5 (38)	3.19 (16)	1.55 (9)	4.48 (34)	4.83 (34)	9.02 (34)	1.53 (39)
Poland	142.2 (23)	103.9 (21)	3.61 (15)	0.98 (19)	7.36 (27)	6.61 (28)	30.16 (22)	7.86 (6)
Portugal	113.6 (32)	84.4 (33)	4.71 (7)	0.96 (20)	11.80 (22)	11.66 (19)	10.91 (33)	2.74 (36)
Rumania	121.1 (31)	87.1 (31)	2.71 (22)	0.78 (27)	5.94 (30)	5.65 (30)	25.86 (24)	5.12 (21)
Scotland	202.8 (1)	124.6 (6)	3.77 (13)	1.58 (8)	24.77 (1)	20.87 (1)	78.14 (1)	11.71 (2)
South Africa	171.0 (10)	113.4 (13)	6.11 (5)	1.16 (14)	1.47 (39)	1.44 (39)	37.63 (13)	6.93 (11)
Sweden	126.1 (27)	104.5 (20)	2.27 (26)	1.33 (12)	16.12 (16)	12.80 (17)	17.35 (27)	4.34 (27)
Switzerland	164.4 (13)	107.6 (17)	6.31 (4)	0.85 (23)	18.91 (11)	13.23 (16)	37.33 (16)	3.33 (34)
Venezuela	105.2 (33)	109.2 (15)	2.92 (19)	3.35 (2)	5.91 (31)	5.49 (31)	1.75 (32)	4.09 (28)
Yugoslavia	102.4 (34)	73.3 (36)	1.85 (30)	0.48 (39)	5.78 (32)	5.24 (32)	23.23 (25)	4.16 (26)

* Figures in parentheses are order of rank within site and sex group.

TABLE 10—continued

Country	Breast Female	Uterus Female	Skin Male	Skin Female	Stomach Male	Stomach Female	Prostate Male	Leukemia Male	Leukemia Female
United States	21.83 (9)	10.85 (22)	2.51 (4)	1.47 (18)	9.5 (38)	4.7 (37)	13.82 (10)	7.49 (4)	4.81 (7)
Australia	19.15 (14)	8.28 (33)	4.42 (1)	2.64 (2)	15.4 (34)	7.7 (35)	13.98 (9)	6.27 (16)	4.45 (16)
Austria	17.47 (18)	17.67 (8)	2.02 (11)	1.60 (12)	40.0 (3)	22.3 (5)	13.38 (12)	5.66 (21)	4.58 (11)
Belgium	20.97 (12)	12.19 (13)	1.80 (20)	1.10 (29)	25.7 (19)	13.8 (18)	15.36 (6)	6.14 (19)	4.20 (22)
Bulgaria	8.75 (29)	7.35 (35)	1.53 (26)	1.18 (27)	37.6 (8)	22.9 (3)	6.15 (32)	4.89 (28)	3.75
Canada	23.47 (4)	10.37 (26)	1.85 (17)	1.30 (29)	16.0 (32)	7.6 (36)	13.16 (14)	6.77 (9)	4.40 (18)
Chile	9.37 (27)	20.09 (3)	1.00 (32)	0.95 (31)	55.6 (2)	32.7 (2)	9.48 (24)	3.95 (31)	3.08 (31)
China	3.72 (36)	15.62 (11)	1.71 (22)	1.15 (27)	18.4 (29)	12.3 (23)	1.07 (39)	2.39 (37)	1.83 (37)
Colombia	5.55 (34)	20.11 (2)	1.25 (30)	1.11 (28)	27.9 (15)	20.4 (8)	5.63 (34)	3.13 (36)	2.28 (35)
Czechoslovakia	14.94 (22)	11.68 (21)	2.28 (8)	1.76 (8)	39.5 (6)	20.7 (7)	8.86 (26)	6.40 (14)	4.34 (19)
Denmark	24.62 (3)	16.66 (9)	1.99 (12)	1.70 (9)	20.6 (26)	10.8 (27)	12.84 (16)	8.13 (2)	4.56 (13)
Dominican Rep.	2.90 (37)	6.76 (37)	0.51 (36)	0.45 (37)	3.8 (39)	1.5 (39)	3.74 (36)	0.92 (39)	1.06 (39)
England & Wales	24.58 (2)	9.68 (28)	1.52 (28)	1.19 (26)	22.7 (25)	10.5 (29)	11.98 (19)	5.49 (22)	3.82 (24)
Finland	14.65 (23)	9.45 (29)	2.13 (10)	1.58 (15)	35.6 (9)	18.5 (12)	11.34 (20)	6.75 (10)	4.88 (6)
France	16.98 (19)	10.62 (24)	1.81 (19)	1.33 (19)	19.2 (27)	9.6 (31)	15.05 (7)	6.53 (12)	4.51 (14)
Germany (F.R.)	18.03 (16)	12.81 (13)	1.98 (13)	1.57 (16)	33.3 (11)	18.5 (11)	5.82 (33)	6.01 (20)	4.44 (15)
Greece	8.19 (32)	5.92 (38)	0.95 (33)	0.89 (32)	14.7 (35)	8.7 (33)	2.35 (37)	7.33 (6)	4.78 (9)
Hong Kong	8.42 (31)	12.41 (17)	0.94 (34)	0.46 (36)	15.6 (33)	10.2 (28)	13.16 (15)	3.39 (35)	3.19 (29)
Hungary	14.57 (24)	18.26 (7)	1.90 (14)	1.59 (13)	40.6 (5)	22.5 (4)	15.47 (4)	6.26 (18)	4.40 (17)
Iceland	18.14 (17)	19.68 (4)	0.43 (38)	3.09 (1)	38.7 (7)	20.1 (9)	12.10 (18)	8.69 (1)	4.62 (10)
Ireland	21.03 (11)	8.10 (34)	2.41 (7)	2.33 (5)	23.6 (22)	15.6 (16)	7.24 (30)	5.18 (25)	3.42 (28)
Israel	21.48 (10)	4.96 (39)	1.46 (29)	1.62 (11)	17.4 (30)	11.2 (26)	9.29 (25)	7.44 (5)	5.76 (1)
Italy	16.09 (21)	12.54 (16)	1.58 (24)	1.06 (30)	31.3 (14)	16.9 (14)	1.82 (38)	6.55 (11)	4.57 (12)
Japan	3.99 (39)	12.72 (15)	0.79 (34)	0.62 (35)	65.4 (1)	34.3 (1)	4.33 (35)	3.82 (34)	2.96 (34)
Mexico	4.18 (36)	19.42 (5)	0.54 (35)	0.84 (33)	10.1 (37)	8.8 (32)	14.69 (8)	2.21 (38)	1.90 (36)
Netherlands	26.45 (1)	10.07 (27)	1.54 (25)	1.27 (24)	26.5 (16)	14.2 (17)	13.67 (11)	7.18 (7)	5.03 (5)
New Zealand	23.11 (5)	9.44 (30)	3.38 (3)	2.57 (3)	16.4 (31)	7.8 (34)	10.70 (22)	6.27 (17)	5.23 (2)
Northern Ireland	20.67 (13)	6.96 (36)	1.89 (15)	1.34 (20)	23.2 (23)	12.3 (22)	16.06 (3)	5.28 (24)	3.69 (26)
Norway	16.78 (20)	9.12 (31)	2.46 (5)	1.63 (10)	25.2 (18)	13.5 (20)	10.16 (23)	7.00 (8)	5.17 (3)
Panama	8.50 (30)	14.66 (12)	1.81 (18)	0.37 (38)	13.8 (36)	5.6 (38)	7.83 (28)	3.88 (32)	1.57 (38)
Poland	10.97 (26)	16.02 (10)	1.75 (21)	1.58 (14)	40.9 (4)	19.4 (10)	8.60 (27)	5.15 (26)	3.60 (27)
Portugal	11.93 (25)	12.73 (14)	1.61 (23)	1.29 (23)	32.2 (13)	17.0 (13)	7.70 (29)	5.33 (23)	4.16 (23)
Rumania	8.89 (28)	19.40 (6)	1.14 (31)	0.79 (34)	31.7 (12)	16.0 (15)	12.15 (17)	4.44 (29)	3.17 (30)
Scotland	22.80 (7)	10.44 (25)	1.48 (28)	1.52 (17)	25.9 (17)	12.7 (21)	19.51 (1)	5.00 (27)	4.31 (21)
South Africa	23.11 (6)	12.18 (19)	3.46 (2)	2.41 (4)	23.8 (21)	11.4 (25)	17.09 (2)	7.87 (3)	4.80 (8)
Sweden	18.00 (15)	9.05 (32)	1.87 (16)	1.32 (21)	19.8 (28)	10.6 (30)	15.46 (5)	6.46 (13)	5.06 (4)
Switzerland	22.15 (8)	11.82 (20)	2.45 (6)	1.80 (7)	24.4 (20)	13.6 (19)	11.01 (21)	6.32 (15)	4.34 (20)
Venezuela	8.02 (34)	27.03 (1)	2.16 (9)	2.07 (6)	34.6 (10)	21.5 (6)	15.46 (5)	3.87 (33)	3.06 (33)
Yugoslavia	8.12 (33)	10.71 (23)	1.54 (27)	1.21 (25)	22.3 (24)	11.7 (24)	6.31 (31)	4.37 (30)	3.07 (32)

TABLE 11
A Condensed Outline of the National Cancer Program

PREVENTION

1. Develop the means to reduce the effectiveness of external agents in producing cancer.
   A. Detect and identify external carcinogenic agents.
   B. Determine human relevance of external carcinogenic agents.
   C. Modify host response to carcinogenic agents, including metabolism of chemical carcinogens, to reduce rate of cancer development.
   D. Improve animal models of human cancer and evaluate the effects of combined factors.
   E. Apply current knowledge and develop (immediately) applicable information.

2. Develop the means to modify individuals in order to minimize the risk of cancer development.
   A. Reduce development of cancer by altering immunological capability of individuals.
   B. Alter metabolism of individuals to reduce rate of cancer development.
   C. Alter genetic makeup or gene expression to reduce the rate of cancer development.
   D. Remove or alter precancerous metabolic or structural lesions.
   E. Identify groups at increased risk of cancer due to or associated with genetic or behavioral factors.
   F. Determine groups at risk of cancer to indicate which individuals might be identified for special preventative help; indicate means for cancer risk modifications and evaluations.

3. Develop the means to prevent transformation of normal cells to cells capable of causing cancer.
   A. Study the nature and modification of the precancerous state and determine mechanisms accounting for high degrees of stability of cell functioning.
   B. Delineate the nature and rate of oncogenic cell transformations in carcinogenesis (including aspects of cell culture and viruses).
   C. Investigate cellular and organismal modifiers of the transformation and promotion processes.
   D. Identify immunological aspects of transformation.
   E. Study cell surfaces and cell membranes.

4. Develop the means to prevent the progression of precancerous cells to cancers, the development of cancers from precancerous conditions, and the spread of cancers from primary sites.
   A. Investigate the biology of cells already capable of forming cancer to determine the relationship between their growth and interaction with the host response.
   B. Develop methods for detecting, locating, and following microfoci of cancer cells and interfere with the advancement of microfoci to clinically significant cancers.
   C. Interfere with the process of tumor initiation following cell transformation, including interference with development of stromal and blood vessel elements and other host responses.
   D. Develop mathematical models of the cancerous process, with emphasis on those steps preceding and following cell transformation.

DETECTION, DIAGNOSIS, PROGNOSIS

5. Develop the means to achieve an accurate assessment of (a) the risk of developing cancer in individuals and in population groups and (b) the presence, extent, and probable course of existing cancers.
   A. Identity population groups with high and low risks of developing cancer.
   B. Identify precancerous lesions and other states associated with cancer.
   C. Extend and improve procedures for screening of population groups.
   D. Improve diagnostic procedures for cancer and for localization of lesions.
   E. Determine (predict) which individuals will eventually get cancer.
   F. Determine characteristics of cancer that produce different growth rates and probabilities of dissemination.
   G. Develop measures for public acceptance and use of preventive measures, screening, and detection methods.

TREATMENT

6. Develop the means to cure cancer patients and to control the progress of cancer.
   A. Develop and utilize methodologies of immunology, chemotherapy, surgery, and irradiation (alone and in combinations) in the cure and palliation of cancer.
   B. Discover new therapeutic agents and develop means for their selection.
   C. Reverse cell transformation from cancer to noncancer (modification of cell control mechanisms by changing kinetics of metabolism and biochemistry, patterns of messenger RNA's, modification of transcription, etc.).
   D. Enhance the host's ability to eliminate or prevent further development of cancer.
   E. Extend research knowledge to all patients (public information, professional education, development of resources).
   F. Develop an epidemiology of treatment (i.e., determine which groups of patients are likely to benefit from specific types of treatment).

REHABILITATION

7. Develop the means to improve the rehabilitation of cancer patients.
   A. Increase the national capacity to provide rehabilitative services for cancer patients.
   B. Develop improved means to provide totally integrated rehabilitative treatment to the cancer patient.

TABLE 12
The Seven Warning Signals of Cancer
[Source: American Cancer Society]

Changing bowel or bladder habits
A sore that does not heal
Unusual bleeding or discharge
Thickening or lump in breast or elsewhere
Indigestion or difficulty in swallowing
Obvious change in wart or mole
Nagging cough or hoarseness

Glossary

On the following pages are defined some of the terms encountered most frequently in discussing cancer. The primary emphasis is on words used in the main text, but many other terms are included. The list is by no means exhaustive, but it should provide a brief introduction to most of the key concepts in cancer research.

Words in italics within a definition (except the Latin names of species) are defined elsewhere in the glossary.

Actinomycin D   Also known as dactinomycin. An antitumor *antibiotic* originally isolated from *Streptomyces parvulus*. It binds tightly to cellular DNA to inhibit the synthesis of RNA.

Adenocarcinoma   A malignant *tumor* of epithelial cells in which the cells are arranged in the form of a gland.

Adenoma   A benign *tumor* of epithelial cells in which the cells are arranged in the form of a gland.

Adenoviruses   DNA *viruses* that cause diseases of the upper respiratory tract. They are also present in a latent form in many healthy individuals. The *genome* of adenoviruses has a mass of 23×10^6 daltons. Some 28 different types of adenoviruses have been identified, and several of them have been shown to produce *tumors* in laboratory animals or to *transform* cultured cells.

Adjuvant chemotherapy   The use of chemotherapy in conjunction with surgery, radiotherapy, or both to try to ensure that all *tumor* cells are killed at the time of treatment. This approach is based on the principles (1) that chemotherapy is most effective when there are only a small number of malignant cells to be dealt with and (2) that surgery and radiotherapy often leave a small number of undiscerned malignant cells.

Adrenal glands   Two small organs, located next to the kidneys, that are responsible for the synthesis and release of several *hormones*, primarily catecholamines and *steroids*.

Adriamycin   An antitumor *antibiotic* isolated from a mutant strain of *Streptomyces peucetius*. It is believed to act by binding with cellular DNA to block the production of RNA. Adriamycin is an analog of *daunorubicin*.

Aflatoxin   A very powerful, naturally occurring carcinogen produced by some strains of a mold, *Aspergillus flavus,* that grows on damp peanuts and other crops.

Agglutination   The clumping together of cells suspended in a fluid in response to the binding of an external agent to appropriate receptors on the cell surface. Malignant cells in culture, for example, agglutinate in the presence of *lectins.*

Alkylating agents   Antitumor agents that can donate an alkyl group to another molecule. The antitumor alkylating agents are usually, but not always, polyfunctional. One way in which they are thought to act is by cross-linking cellular DNA, thereby interfering with its ability to be replicated and to serve as a template for the synthesis of RNA. Some alkylating agents are carcinogenic.

Alpha-fetoprotein (AFP)   A protein that occurs in the blood of normal embryos and infants and of adults with liver *tumors.* Its presence in adults was originally thought to be specific for the presence of a liver tumor, but it has subsequently been observed in individuals with a few other types of tumors or with liver diseases such as hepatitis. It has also been found in higher than normal concentrations in pregnant women who subsequently bore children with certain types of congenital abnormalities.

Alpha particle   The nucleus of a helium atom; that is, a particle containing two protons and two neutrons. There is evidence to suggest that alpha particles may be useful in the radiotherapy of *tumors.*

Allergy   A pathological reactivity to antigens, manifested by excessive sneezing, difficult breathing, itching, or skin rashes.

Amethopterin   *Methotrexate.*

Aminopterin   4-Aminopteroyl glutamic acid. A *folic acid* analog that acts as an *antimetabolite* in the same fashion as *methotrexate.*

Anaplasia A structural abnormality, characteristic of *tumor* cells, in which cells resemble more primitive or embryonic cells and in which adult cell functions are absent or diminished. Anaplastic cells also lack orientation with respect to the parent tissue; instead of an orderly spatial arrangement, their distribution is generally jumbled.

Androgens *Hormones* that produce the physical characteristics of the male. The primary adrogen of humans is testosterone, which is synthesized in the testes.

Angioma A benign *tumor* arising in cells from blood vessels (hemangioma) or from *lymph* vessels (lymphangioma).

Angiosarcoma A *sarcoma* that contains very many small blood vessels.

Antibiotics Complex, naturally-occurring compounds, produced by microbial fermentation, which inhibit the growth of microorganisms. Some possess antitumor properties. Some of these, such as *actinomycin D* and *Adriamycin* bind to cellular DNA, thereby preventing its transcription. The mechanism of action of some others is unknown.

Antibody A complex protein (immunoglobulin) synthesized by certain types of *lymphocytes* in response to an *antigen*. Antibodies have two or more specific sites complementary in structure to groupings on the antigen so that they can combine with it. If the antigen is part of a cell, attachment of the antibody to the antigen in the presence of appropriate accessory factors, such as *complement,* may lead to eventual destruction of the cell.

Antigen Also called an immunogen. A high–molecular weight substance, usually a protein or a complex of protein and polysaccharide, that stimulates the formation of specific *antibodies* or specific *lymphocytes* in an animal to which it is foreign.

Antimetabolites Chemicals that have a close structural resemblance to normal metabolites. Antimetabolites either substitute for a normal metabolite to block crucial enzymes or otherwise interfere with the metabolism of cells. In some cases, antimetabolites are preferentially toxic to *tumor* cells and can be used as antitumor agents.

Among the best known antimetabolites active against tumors are *methotrexate* and *5-fluorouracil.*

Arabinosyl cytosine   Also known as cytosine arabinoside, cytarabine, or Ara-C. An *antimetabolite* of cytidylic acid in which the sugar arabinose is substituted for the sugar ribose, the normal sugar in RNA. It substitutes for cytidylic acid to inhibit the enzyme that converts cytidylic acid to deoxycytidylic acid and also inhibits DNA polymerase; in both cases, it inhibits the biosynthesis of DNA. It is especially useful for treatment of acute *leukemias.*

Aryl hydrocarbon hydroxylases (AHH's)   A family of enzymes, found in *microsomes,* that can add a hydroxyl group—possibly through an intermediary epoxide—to *polycyclic aromatic hydrocarbons* such as benzo[*a*]pyrene.

L-*Asparaginase*   An enzyme that hydrolyzes the amino acid asparagine into aspartic acid and ammonia. Certain types of *tumor* cells, especially in *leukemias,* require an external source of asparagine. Bacterial or animal L-asparaginase administered intravenously thus acts as an antitumor agent by reducing the aspargine content of body fluids.

Autoimmune disease   A disorder in which an individual's immune system attacks his own healthy tissues. Arthritis, for example, is believed by many investigators to be an autoimmune disease.

Avian leukosis-sarcoma viruses   A family of *type C RNA viruses* that cause malignant diseases in fowl, especially chickens. The *Rous sarcoma virus* is an example.

5-Azacytidine An antitumor *antimetabolite* that is incorporated into RNA. Its exact mechanism of action is not known.

Azathioprine Also known as Immuran. A derivative of the *antimetabolite 6-mercaptopurine* that is thought to act as an antitumor agent by releasing 6-mercaptopurine inside *tumor* cells, probably through a reaction with sulfhydryl compounds.

Bacillus Calmette-Guérin (BCG) An attenuated strain of the bacterium, Mycobacterium bovis, that causes bovine tuberculosis. It is frequently used as a vaccine against human tuberculosis (especially in Europe) and is generally thought to be a potent nonspecific stimulator of the immune system. It is thus sometimes used on an experimental basis for the treatment of *tumors.*

Basal cell carcinoma A skin *tumor* that in many respects appears to be intermediate between a benign and a malignant tumor. Basal cell *carcinomas* invade, compress, and destroy surrounding tissues and erode through bone and cartilage, but almost never *metastasize.*

Basophil A type of *granulocyte* that accounts for about 0.5 percent of *leukocytes* in the blood. Basophils are chemically, structurally, and functionally similar to the *mast cells* found in connective tissues.

They contain large amounts of heparin and vasoamines (histamine, serotonin, dopamine). Their primary physiological function is unknown, but their distribution suggests that they help regulate the permeability of terminal blood vessel nets by release of the vaso- amines. Abnormal release of these amines contributes to the *inflammation* observed in *hypersensitivity* and in some non- immunological disorders.

BCG   *Bacillus Calmette-Guérin.*

BCNU   A *nitrosourea* used as an *alkylating agent* in the treatment of tumors.

$$Cl-CH_2CH_2-N-\overset{\overset{\displaystyle O}{\|}}{C}-NH-CH_2CH_2-Cl$$
$$\underset{N=O}{|}$$

Bence-Jones protein   A low-molecular weight, temperature-sensitive urinary protein that is found in patients with *multiple myeloma.* It is a fragment of immunoglobulin molecules. It has the unique prop- erty of coagulating when heated to 45 to 55°C and redissolving either partially or wholly when further heated to boiling.

Benign tumor   See *tumor.*

Biopsy   The surgical removal of a small piece of tissue for laboratory examination by a pathologist to determine if it is malignant.

Bittner virus   *Mouse mammary tumor virus.*

Bleomycin   A mixture of antitumor *antibiotics* isolated from *Strep- tomyces verticillus.* Present data suggest that the primary action of the bleomycins is the scission of DNA strands or the inhibition of a DNA ligase (repair enzyme) with resultant inhibition of cell division and production of fatally damaged daughter cells. Bleomy- cins are among the few antitumor agents that do not depress synthesis of *lymphocytes* in *bone marrow.*

Blocking factor   An unidentified substance, found in the blood serum of animals with growing *tumors,* that will block the action of *immune lymphocytes* previously sensitized to that tumor. The activity of blocking factor has been demonstrated primarily with cultured tumor cells. Many investigators think blocking factor is a complex of tumor *antigen* and host *antibody.*

B lymphocyte Also known as thymus-independent lymphocyte or bursa-equivalent lymphocyte. A type of *lymphocyte*, accounting for 20 to 30 percent of lymphocytes in the blood, that is involved in *humoral immunity*, synthesis of *antibodies*, and immediate *hypersensitivity* reactions. B lymphocyte precursors originate in *bone marrow* (and perhaps also in other lymphoid tissues). They either are distributed directly to the spleen, *lymph nodes*, and other lymphoid tissues or are processed by the spleen, intestines, or tonsils to become mature, functional B lymphocytes. In addition to circulating in the blood, B lymphocytes are also found in the germinal centers of lymph nodes, the gastrointestinal tract, secretory glands, *bone marrow*, the appendix, and other lymphoid tissues associated with the *reticuloendothelial system.* B lymphocytes are precursors of plasma cells, the form that actually secretes *antibodies.*

Bone marrow Soft tissues in the medullary canals of long bones and in the interstices of cancellous (spongy) bone. Bone marrow is the primary site for production of *leukocytes* and is thus an important constituent of the body's immune system.

Bone marrow grafts A technique sometimes used in the treatment of myelocytic *leukemias.* To ensure that all leukemia cells are destroyed, all the patient's *bone marrow* cells are killed by drugs or radiation. This treatment leaves the patient highly susceptible to infectious diseases, however, so some physicians have attempted to transplant healthy bone marrow cells from a carefully matched donor to provide immune protection for the patient. This technique has been successful only to a limited extent, in part because the patients often die from infections before the grafted cells begin functioning, and in part because the donor cells often mount an immune reaction against the patient. The latter phenomenon is known as graft-versus-host disease.

Bragg peak A sharp increase in the radiation energy transferred to a tissue by a charged particle as the particle comes to a halt. If the initial energy of such a particle is adjusted properly, the particle will come to rest in an internal *tumor* and most of the radiation will be released to the tumor.

Bromodeoxyuridine (BUDR) A *nucleoside* analog that can function as an *antimetabolite* by substituting for thymidine in DNA synthesis.

Its common effect is interference with the *differentiation* of cells. It is frequently used for the induction of *latent viruses* in cultured cells. It is also a *mutagen.*

Bronchogenic carcinoma A malignant *tumor* of the lung.

Burkitt's lymphoma A *tumor* of the lymphoid system that arises in facial bones, ovaries, and abdominal *lymph nodes.* It is the most common tumor of children in certain parts of Africa and New Guinea, but it is seldom observed in the United States and Western Europe. It is thought to be caused by the *Epstein–Barr virus,* but the evidence is not conclusive.

Busulfan An *alkylating agent* used for the treatment of *tumors.*

Cachexia The generalized emaciation of an ill individual, particularly a cancer patient, resulting from severe malnutrition. The malnutrition of cancer patients results not only from the failure of the patient to consume food, but also from a malignant tumor's unexplained priority on nutrients within the host; the tumor nourishes itself at the expense of healthy tissues.

Capsid The protein layer surrounding the nucleic acid core of a *virus.*

Carcinoembryonic antigen (CEA) A glycoprotein originally isolated from colon *tumors* and subsequently found in fetal tissues. Its function is not yet known. CEA was at first thought to be a unique marker for colon tumors in adults, but more recent studies have shown that it is present in small quantities in normal blood and is present in increased amounts in the blood of smokers, of individuals with emphysema or cirrhosis of the liver, and of individuals with certain other types of tumors.

Carcinogen   Any agent that initiates the formation of a *tumor*.

Carcinoma   A malignant *tumor* arising in epithelial tissues. These include skin, glands, nerves, breasts, and the linings of the respiratory, gastrointestinal, urinary, and genital systems. Carcinomas account for about 85 percent of human malignancies.

Carcinoma-in-situ   Also known as preinvasive *carcinoma*. A type of *tumor* in which the abnormal cells still lie within the *epithelium* of origin, without invasion of the basement membrane. The term is often applied to such tumors in the uterine cervix. Because the tumor is localized, the survival rate after its removal is very high.

Carminomycin   An antitumor *antibiotic* that is thought to act by binding to DNA to block the production of RNA. It is a synthetically prepared analog of *daunorubicin*.

CCNU   Also known as Lomustine. A *nitrosourea* used as an *alkylating* agent in the treatment of *tumors*.

Cell-mediated immunity   The system that is responsible for primary rejection of transplants, delayed *hypersensitivity*, surveillance against *tumors,* and protection against viruses and bacteria. Sensitized *T lymphocytes* in contact with target *antigens* release a number of factors that act against the foreign substance. These include: mitogenic factor, a nonspecific substance which is thought to stimulate proliferation of previously quiescent *lymphocytes;* *migration inhibition factor,* which causes *macrophages* to be retained in the area of the foreign material; lymphotoxin, a substance released by sensitized lymphocytes for the destruction of target cells such as those of a tumor or bacteria; *transfer factor;* chemotactic factor, which attracts macrophages and *granulocytes* to the area of inflammation; and interferon, an agent that acts against viruses. Most of these substances have not been characterized chemically and their mechanisms of action are understood only to a limited extent.

Chlorambucil   Also known as Leukeran. An *alkylating agent* used in the treatment of *tumors.*

$$(ClCH_2CH_2)_2-N-\langle\!\!\bigcirc\!\!\rangle-CH_2CH_2CH_2COOH$$

Chondroma   A benign *tumor* arising in cartilage (a tissue that lines joints and is present at the growing end of bones).

Chondrosarcoma   A malignant *tumor* arising in cartilage (a tissue that lines joints and is present at the growing end of bones).

Choriocarcinoma   A malignant *tumor* arising in the *epithelium* of the placenta.

Chromosomes   Structures containing the cell's nuclear DNA. During cell division (*mitosis*), these structures become compacted into heavily staining, rod-shaped bodies that are easily seen under the microscope. Each species has a characteristic number of chromosomes; in man, that number is 46.

Citrovorum factor   A *folic acid* derivative that is identical to or substitutes for the product of the enzyme folic acid reductase. If that enzyme has been inhibited by an *antimetabolite,* such as *methotrexate,* administration of citrovorum factor enables the cell to bypass the inhibited enzyme. For some reason, citrovorum factor works more effectively in healthy cells than in malignant ones, so its use means that higher doses of methotrexate can be administered to treat *tumors.*

Clinical trial The systematic investigation of materials or methods, according to a formal study plan, as a means of determining effect or relative effectiveness in a human population with a particular disease or class of diseases. In clinical trials of therapeutic methods, the choice of therapeutic protocol is typically random so that neither the patient nor the clinician knows if the patient is receiving the protocol to be tested, an accepted protocol that serves as a control, or a placebo protocol that is, in effect, no treatment at all.

Cobalt-60 A radioactive isotope of the element cobalt that is used as a source of *gamma rays* in the radiotherapy of *tumors.*

Colony-stimulating factor (CSF) An unidentified *glycoprotein,* isolated from blood, that will apparently induce cultured *lymphocytes* from patients with acute myelocytic *leukemia* to mature. The relation of this factor to the disease process in vivo is still undetermined.

Colostomy The surgical creation of a new opening of the colon on the surface of the body. The term is sometimes incorrectly used to refer to the stoma, the opening itself.

Combination chemotherapy The simultaneous use of several antitumor agents to treat a malignancy. This approach is based on the principle that, with judicious selection of drugs, the antitumor effects will be at least additive while the toxic effects will not.

Complement A group of 11 serum proteins that interact sequentially with certain *antigen-antibody* complexes. If the antigen is part of a cell, this interaction may lead to destruction of that cell.

Contact inhibition Also known as density-dependent inhibition of growth. The phenomenon in which healthy cells growing in culture stop dividing and become immobilized once they have formed a contiguous monolayer covering the surface of the substrate on which they grow. Loss of contact inhibition is one measure of *transformation.*

Cyclic AMP (cAMP) Adenosine-3′,5′-monophosphate, a widely dispersed chemical whose primary function is believed to be the mediation of *hormone* action. Some hormones act, at least in part, by initiating the synthesis of cAMP in the target cells. cAMP thus acts like an intracellular hormone, and hence is often called "the second messenger." Changes in cAMP concentrations have been associated with, among other things, mobilization of substrates for enzymes, release of hormones, changes in the permeability of the cell membrane, sensory and neural excitation, and *transformation* of cultured cells.

Cyclophosphamide   Also known as Cytoxan. An *alkylating agent* used in the treatment of *tumors.*

Cyclotron   A circular device in which atomic particles are accelerated by an alternating electric field in a constant magnetic field.

Cyst   An accumulation of nonviable material, often fluid, within a body cavity surrounded by a definite wall. The contents of the cavity may be retained normal secretions, as in the obstruction of a glandular duct, or fluids associated with a parasitic infection.

Cytoplasm   The usually jellylike mass that fills the space between the external membrane of a cell's nucleus and the membrane that delimits the cell. It is composed of water and a wide variety of chemical substances, some of which are organized into small structures (organelles) which perform specific cellular functions.

Cytosine arabinoside   *Arabinosyl cytosine.*

Daunorubicin Also known as daunomycin. An antitumor *antibiotic* isolated from *Streptomyces peucetius.* It is believed to act by binding to DNA to block the synthesis of RNA.

o,p'-DDD An antitumor agent that is thought to inhibit the production of *steroid hormones.* It is thus useful in the treatment of adrenal carcinoma.

Density-dependent inhibition of growth Contact inhibition.

Dexamethasone A synthetic *steroid hormone* that is often used as an anti-inflammatory or antiallergic agent. It can sometimes be used to induce the appearance of *latent viruses* in cultured cells.

Dibromodulcitol   An *alkylating agent* used in the treatment of *tumors*.

$$
\begin{array}{c}
CH_2-Br \\
H-C-OH \\
HO-C-H \\
HO-C-H \\
H-C-OH \\
CH_2-Br
\end{array}
$$

Dibromomannitol   An *alkylating agent* used in the treatment of *tumors*.

$$
\begin{array}{c}
CH_2-Br \\
HO-C-H \\
HO-C-H \\
H-C-OH \\
H-C-OH \\
CH_2-Br
\end{array}
$$

Differentiation   The act or process of acquiring completely individual character and specific functions, such as occurs in the progressive diversification of cells and tissues in the embryo. The mechanism of differentiation is unknown. Malignancy generally involves a loss of differentiation.

Down's syndrome   Also known as mongolism. A genetic defect characterized by mental retardation, slanting eyes, a broad, short skull, and broad hands with short fingers. The specific genetic lesion in Down's syndrome is the presence of an extra *chromosome* number 21. Children with Down's syndrome have a 15-fold higher incidence of *leukemia* than do normal children.

Effector cells   Small *lymphocytes* ("killer" cells) that recognize and destroy cultured *tumor* cells or other cells to which they are sensitized.

Electrophilic   Electron-deficient; referring to a portion (electrophile or electrophilic center) of a molecule capable of attacking electron-rich (*nucleophilic*) centers in other molecules. Typical electrophilic centers include carbonium ions, free-radicals, epoxides, and some metal cations. Electrophilic centers are believed to be the reactive sites of most, if not all, chemical *carcinogens*.

Endogenous viruses   *Viruses* that are thought to be produced by the expression of a *virogene* in a cell, but that may simply exist in intimate association with cellular DNA. The most common of these are *type C RNA viruses.* Endogenous *xenotropic viruses* are transmitted genetically; they are noninfectious in cells of the species of origin, but are often infectious in cells of other species. Endogenous ecotropic viruses are infectious in cells of the species of origin and may be transmitted by either genetic or *epigenetic* mechanisms. Many scientists now believe that all mammalian and avian cells contain virogenes to produce endogenous viruses, but the physiological function of such viruses is still unknown. Most of the endogenous viruses have not been shown to be *oncogenic.*

Endoscopy   The insertion of an optical instrument into body cavities or passages to the interior—such as the esophagus, trachea, ears, anus, urinary tract, or genital tract—to explore for hidden *tumors* or other abnormalities.

Endothelioma   A malignant *tumor* arising in endothelial cells that line blood vessels and *lymph* vessels.

Eosinophil   A type of *granulocyte* that comprises about 2 to 5 percent of the total *leukocytes* in the blood. *Bone marrow* contains about 200 times more eosinophils than does blood, and some tissues (intestinal walls, skin, external genitalia, lungs) contain as much as 500 times more. Their concentration is regulated by *adrenal hormones.* Eosinophil granules contain many of the same enzymes as do *neutrophils,* with the major exception of lysozyme and phagocytin. The functions of eosinophils are largely unknown, but they do have a limited capability for *phagocytosis.* They may also play a role in allergic reactions.

Epidermoid carcinoma   A malignant *tumor* arising from the skin.

Epigenetic   Referring to an event that produces an apparent change in heredity without a chemical change in the DNA of the *genome.* One such event might be a protein change that leads to a relatively permanent change in the expression of genes.

Epithelioma   A malignant *tumor* consisting mainly of cells from the *epithelium* and primarily derived from the skin or mucous surfaces.

Epithelium The covering of internal and external surfaces of the body, glands, nerves, breasts, and the linings of the respiratory, gastrointestinal, urinary, and genital systems.

Epstein–Barr virus Also known as EB virus. A *herpesvirus* that has been shown to be the cause of infectious mononucleosis and that is thought to be the case of *Burkitt's lymphoma* and some forms of postnasal *carcinoma.*

Ewing's sarcoma A malignant *tumor* arising in *bone marrow.* It occurs most often in cylindrical bones, and the most prominent symptoms are pain, fever, and an increase in the number of *leukocytes* in the blood.

Exfoliative cytology The microscopic examination of cells that have flaked off of (primarily) interior body surfaces to determine if a hidden *tumor* is present. Exfoliative cytology is a very powerful technique for discovering tumors, but it is useful only in those cases where the exfoliated cells can be readily obtained by a physician. The most common application is the *Pap smear*, where the exfoliated cells are from the uterus.

Exogenous viruses *Viruses* that are foreign to the primary host cells. This category includes all viruses except the comparatively small class of *endogenous viruses.*

Fanconi's aplastic anemia A genetic defect in which all blood components show a reduced proliferation. About 10 percent of children with this disorder develop acute monomyelocytic *leukemia,* a rare form that accounts for less than 4 percent of all leukemias.

Fetal antigens Substances (primarily proteins, *glycoproteins,* and polysaccharides) found in health almost exclusively in embryonic tissues and fetuses. They are rather loosely described as *antigens* because of the immune reaction they provoke in laboratory animals and, in most cases, in mature animals of the same species. Many fetal antigens have been observed in adults with malignant *tumors.*

Fibroblast A connective tissue cell. Fibroblasts form the fibrous tissues in the body, such as tendons, and supporting and binding tissues of all sorts.

Fibroma A benign *tumor* of adult connective tissues.

Fibrosarcoma A malignant *tumor* of adult connective tissues.

Fluid mosaic model A hypothetical scheme for the structure of cell membranes. In this model, the surface membranes of cells are dynamic fluid structures in which membrane components may migrate laterally in the membrane plane. This model was proposed to account for the peculiar properties of the membranes of malignant cells, particularly the capability of transformed cultured cells to be *agglutinated* by *lectins*.

5-Fluorouracil An *antimetabolite* that is converted by intracellular enzymes to 5-fluorodeoxyuridine monophosphate. This *nucleotide* inhibits the enzyme thymidylate synthetase, which converts deoxyuridine monophosphate to thymidine monophosphate. 5-Fluorouracil thus inhibits the synthesis of DNA.

Folic acid A vitamin that is, among other things, essential for the transfer of single-carbon fragments in the synthesis of purines for DNA. Folic acid must proceed through two cellular reductions to become tetrahydrofolic acid, which is its active form. Folic acid *antimetabolites* such as *methotrexate* and *aminopterin* block the enzymes that carry out these reductions.

Frameshift mutagen An agent that alters the transcription of DNA by, in effect, either deleting a base from the polymer or inserting an additional one. The most common frameshift *mutagens* are large, planar aromatic hydrocarbons that intercalate between adjacent bases in the DNA double helix so that they are mistaken for an additional base during transcription. The most effective frameshift mutagens have a reactive site so that they can permanently attach themselves to the polymer.

Gamma rays A type of electromagnetic radiation with wavelengths shorter than 10^{-10} meters, shorter than the wavelengths of *x-rays*. Gamma rays thus carry more energy than do x-rays and, when used for radiotherapy, deliver more energy to *tumors*.

Ganglioneuroma A malignant *tumor* arising in adult nerve cells and fibers outside the central nervous system.

Ganglioside A *glycolipid* to which is generally attached at least one mole of *N*-acetylglucosamine or *N*-acetylgalactosamine and at least one mole of *sialic acid*. Globoside, the most abundant ganglioside in the *stroma* of red blood cells, is composed of a glycolipid (ceramide) attached to a molecule of glucose, two molecules of galactose, and one molecule of *N*-acetylgalactosamine. Gangliosides are common components of cellular membranes.

Gene A segment of a cell's DNA (a unit of heredity) that codes for a specific polypeptide. Synthesis of the final gene product is known as expression; if that product is not made, the gene is considered to be repressed.

Gene amplification The occurrence of multiple copies of particular sequences in the *genome* of a cell, that is, multiple copies of a *gene*. Gene amplification is important when large quantities of one type of protein or nucleic acid must be synthesized; it also helps prevent the mutation of a gene from halting production of a crucial enzyme.

Genome The complete set of genetic information passed on to the offspring of a biological entity. In *viruses*, the genome is the entire complement of DNA or RNA. In man and other animals, it is the entire complement of DNA in germ (egg or sperm) cells, and is equal to half the genetic complement of *somatic* cells.

Gibbon ape leukemia virus A *type C RNA virus* that produces *leukemia* in certain primates.

Glioma A generally benign *tumor* arising from several types of specialized connective tissue in the brain and spinal cord.

Glycolipids   Complex molecules containing one or more carbohydrate residues and one or more fatty acids connected by ester or amide linkages. Cerebrosides (illustrated), for example, are fatty acid amides of sphingosine linked to a 6-carbon sugar, generally D-galactose; they are typically found in the brain and other fatty tissues.

$$CH{=}CH{-}\underset{\underset{\displaystyle CH_3}{\overset{\displaystyle (CH_2)_{12}}{|}}}{C}{-}CH_2{-}O$$

Glycolysis   The anaerobic oxidation of glucose to the cellular metabolites pyruvic acid and lactic acid, with the concomitant production of adenosine triphosphate (ATP), the mediator of chemical energy in the cell. Glycolysis is substantially less efficient than aerobic oxidation of glucose. Healthy cells rely primarily on aerobic oxidation; cells of many malignant tumors show a greater degree of glycolysis. This phenomen is known as the *Warburg effect.*

Glycoproteins   Proteins, covalently bound to carbohydrates, in which the sugars comprise less than 4 percent of the molecule's weight. Similar compounds containing more than 4 percent sugars are called mucoproteins.

Granulocytes   A family of leukocytes that accounts for as much as 68 percent of white cells in the blood. The major types of granulocytes are *neutrophils, basophils,* and *eosinophils.*

Granulocytic leukemia   Another term for myelocytic *leukemia.*

Guanazole   An antitumor agent that inhibits the enzyme ribonucleoside diphosphate reductase. It thus blocks the conversion of ribonucleoside diphosphates to their deoxy derivatives, thereby inhibiting the synthesis of DNA.

Hemangioma   A benign *tumor* of the blood vessels.

Hemangiosarcoma   A malignant *tumor* containing both endothelial cells from the linings of blood or lymph vessels and *fibroblasts*.

Hemopoietic cancers   Cancers of the blood-forming organs, that is, *leukemias and lymphomas*.

Hepatoma   A *tumor* of the liver.

Herpes simplex   A family of acute diseases, caused by *herpesviruses*, most commonly marked by groups of watery blisters on the skin and mucous membranes, such as the borders of the lips (herpes labialis) and the mucous membranes of the genitals (herpes genitalis). Disseminated herpes simplex and herpes encephalitis are very serious infections of the newborn.

Herpesviruses   A family of DNA *viruses* that are the cause of, among other things, a group of skin infections known as *herpes simplex* and *herpes zoster*. The DNA of herpesviruses has a mass of about 85 to 100×10^6 daltons. The two major herpesviruses are known as herpes simplex virus I and II (HSV I and II). Herpes simplex virus I is responsible for infections of the mouth, lip (cold sores), cornea, and genital areas, and is thought to be one of the most widely distributed viruses in humans; some 70 to 90 percent of adults are estimated to have antibodies to it. It is transmitted primarily by saliva and by direct contact of healthy skin with fluid from the herpes lesions. Herpes simplex virus II is most frequently responsible for infections of the genital area and is venereally transmitted. Other herpesviruses include *Epstein-Barr virus*, cytomegalovirus, and *herpesvirus saimiri*. Many of the herpesviruses are suspected of being involved in the etiology of *tumors*.

Herpesvirus saimiri   A simian *herpesvirus* that causes *tumors* in certain primates but not in the natural host.

Herpes zoster   A *herpesvirus* that causes chicken pox and herpes zoster (shingles); also the disease called shingles. The latter results from activation of a latent infection and produces eruptions along the paths of nerves in the skin.

Hexamethylmelamine   An *alkylating agent* used in the treatment of tumors.

$$H_3C-N(CH_3)-\text{[triazine ring]}-N(CH_3)-CH_3$$

CH₃ structure:

```
         CH3        CH3
          |          |
  H3C—N    N    N—CH3
         ╲  ╱ ╲  ╱
          N     N
           ╲   ╱
            N
          ╱   ╲
       H3C    CH3
```

Hodgkin's disease   A form of *lymphoma* characterized by progressive, painless enlargement of *lymph nodes*, fever, anemia, and *cachexia*. Enlargement of the lymph nodes is generally accompanied by the presence of characteristic types of *lymphocytes* (Sternberg-Reed cells) and *eosinophils*.

Horizontal transmission   The transfer of a *virus* from one member of a species to another or to a member of another species by postembryonic infection. Horizontal transmission is the normal mode for the spread of many viruses (as opposed to *vertical transmission*), but is apparently uncommon for oncogenic viruses.

Hormone   A chemical substance, produced at certain sites in the body, which has a specific effect on the activity of one or more distant organs.

Humoral immunity   The system, primarily involving *B lymphocytes*, that provides a defense against bacterial and viral infections by the synthesis of specific *antibodies* (immunoglobulins). These antibodies combine with *antigens* of the infectious agent to form complexes that initiate action by other components of the immune system. The humoral immune system is also associated with the phenomenon of immediate *hypersensitivity*—which occurs when a specific immunoglobulin (generally IgE), while bound to a *mast cell*, reacts with an antigen to release substances (notably histamine) that produce characteristic reactions of the skin. Among the other substances associated with immediate hypersensitivity are "slow-reacting substance of anaphylaxis" and serotonin.

Hydroxyurea   An antitumor agent that inhibits the enzyme ribonucleoside diphosphate reductase. It thus blocks the conversion of

ribonucleoside diphosphates to their deoxy derivatives, thereby
inhibiting the synthesis of DNA.

$$H_2N-\underset{\underset{O}{\|}}{C}-NH-OH$$

Hyperplasia   The abnormal proliferation of cells, as in a callus or a
   tumor.

Hypersensitivity   A characteristic reactivity associated with an allergic
   response to an *antigen* (allergen). There are two types: immediate
   hypersensitivity, mediated by the *immunoglobulin* IgE, and delayed
   hypersensitivity, mediated by *lymphocytes.*

Imidazole carboximides   A family of *alkylating agents* used in the
   treatment of *tumors.* One of the most effective is 5-(3,3-dimethyl-1-
   triazeno)imidazole-4-carboxamide. They appear to be especially
   good in the treatment of *melanoma.*

Immune lymphocytes   *Lymphocytes* that have been sensitized by prior
   exposure, either in vivo or in vitro, to *antigens.* Such lymphocytes
   are then able to mount an immune response against cells, including
   tumor cells, to which they were sensitized.

Immune RNA   A type of RNA, extracted from lymphoid tissues, that
   some scientists suggest can transfer *cell-mediated immunity* from
   one individual to another. Its effects are claimed to be *tumor-*
   specific but not species-specific, so that RNA from an immunized
   animal donor could theoretically transfer tumor immunity to
   human patients. It has received only very limited testing in humans.

Immunoglobulins   A group of proteins in blood serum that is part of
   the *humoral immunity* system. In man, there are five classes of
   immunoglobulins: IgG, IgM, IgA, IgF, and IgD. *Antibody* activity is
   characteristic of immunoglobulins.

Immunological surveillance   A hypothetical process in which it is
   postulated that malignant cells continually arise in complex

organisms, such as man, but normally are efficiently detected and eliminated by the organism's immune system. A *tumor* would thus occur when one such cell escapes detection and proliferates without hindrance.

Induction The synthesis of enzymes initiated by exposure of a cell to the enzymes' normal substrates, analogs of the substrates, and sometimes to apparently unrelated chemicals. The phenomenon is particularly apparent in the synthesis of *microsomal mixed-function oxidases* following exposure of certain cells to foreign chemicals.

Inflammation The response of the body to infection or irritation; it is characterized by redness, heat, swelling, and pain. Redness and heat are the result of increased blood supply to the area. Swelling results from loss of blood plasma to the tissue spaces, which compresses nerve endings and causes pain. *Leukocytes* also crowd the tissue space for *phagocytosis* of bacteria or cellular debris and to wall off the infection in order to prevent its spread. As the inflammation subsides, repair of the damaged tissue begins.

Integration The insertion of the *genome* of a DNA *virus*, or of a DNA copy of the genome of an RNA virus, into the genome of a host cell. Such an insertion permits the virus to remain dormant (latent) in the host cell for long periods of time. It also permits transmission of the virus to daughter cells without the appearance of viral proteins or fully assembled viruses that might trigger the host's immune defenses. Much evidence indicates that integration may be a prerequisite for *transformation* of cells by oncogenic viruses.

Iododeoxyuridine (IUDR) A *nucleoside* analog, much like *bromodeoxyuridine.* It is used as an antiviral agent and for the *induction* of *latent viruses* in cultured cells.

Isoenzymes   Also called isozymes. Enzymes that catalyze the same chemical reaction, but which have different kinetic properties (such as ability to bind substrates, maximum velocity of reaction, and so forth) and generally a different but similar amino acid composition. Families of isoenzymes generally have characteristic distribution patterns in tissues at different stages in their embryologic and later development. Isoenzymes may have evolved to meet differing needs for a particular chemical reaction in various tissues or to protect the cell from mutational loss of a crucial enzyme.

Isophosphamide   An *alkylating agent* used in the treatment of *tumors.*

Koch's postulates   Also known as the law of specificity of bacteria. A set of conditions that must be fulfilled before a microorganism (bacterial or viral) can be considered to be the proved cause of a disease. The microorganisms: (1) must be present in every case of the disease; (2) must be isolated and grown in pure culture; (3) must produce the disease when the cultured product is injected into susceptible healthy animals; and (4) [added to Koch's original three postulates by later scientists] must be recovered from the animal thus infected and again grown in culture.

Krebiozen   A white powder "chemically separated from horses' serum after stimulation of their cell network by the injection of *Actinomyces bovis*" that has been used in the treatment of *tumors.* It has been identified by the Food and Drug Administration as creatine, and its use has been discredited.

Laetrile   *l*-Mandelonitrile-β-glucuronic acid. A putative antitumour agent whose activity is said to depend on scission of the molecule at the tumor site by β-glucuronidase to produce hydrogen cyanide, benzaldehyde, and glucuronic acid. Its use has been largely discredited.

Laminar air-flow bedrooms Hospital rooms equipped with fans and air purification systems that create a pattern of air flow such that infectious microorganisms are swept away from a susceptible patient and filtered from the air.

Lapin virus A putative human *leukemia* virus isolated by Boris Lapin of the Soviet Union. It is a *type C RNA virus*. The possibility that it is a human virus has not been corroborated in the United States.

Latent virus A *virus* which cannot be isolated in an infectious form and which is not demonstrable in a cell except by indirect methods or by activation.

Lectins A general term for blood group-specific and *tumor*-specific agglutins that occur in seeds and other parts of certain plants.

Leiomyoma A benign *tumor* arising in smooth muscle tissues.

Leukemia A systemic cancer in which abnormal *leukocytes* accumulate in the blood and *bone marrow*. There are four main types of leukemia; acute and chronic lymphocytic leukemia and acute and chronic myelocytic leukemia. There is some evidence to suggest that acute lymphocytic leukemia is a disorder of *T lymphocytes* and chronic lymphocytic leukemia a disorder of *B lymphocytes*. The myelocytic leukemias are disorders of *granulocytes*, but there is no evidence to suggest a biochemical distinction between the acute and chronic forms. The acute leukemias appear suddenly and progress rapidly; death generally occurs at a median of 3 months without treatment. The chronic leukemias progress much more slowly and the life expectancy is about 3 years.

Leukocytes White blood cells. Leukocytes number about 5000 to 10,000 per cubic millimeter of blood in healthy individuals, as compared to about 4.5 to 5 million erythrocytes (red blood cells) in the same volume. There are two main types of leukocytes: monomorphonuclear and polymorphonuclear. Monomorphonuclear cells, which include *lymphocytes* and *monocytes*, have a large, round or kidney-shaped nucleus. Polymorphonuclear cells, also called myeloid cells, have a lobed nucleus. When polymorphonuclear cells are stained with certain dyes, tiny granules are observed in the cytoplasm; hence, they are also known as *granulocytes*. Granulocytes are subdivided into three main groups: *neutrophils*, *basophils*, and *eosinophils*, according to the color of the granules after staining with a certain dye (Wright's stain). Neutrophils account for 55 to 65 percent of leukocytes in the blood; eosinophils, 1 to 3 percent; basophils, 0 to 0.75 percent; lymphocytes, 25 to 33 percent; and monocytes, 3 to 7 percent.

Leukosis   The abnormal proliferation of tissues that produce *leukocytes*. The term includes myelosis, certain forms of *reticuloendotheliosis*, and lymphadenosis.

Leukovirus   A term used by the International Committee for Nomenclature to categorize RNA tumor viruses. Many virologists prefer and use the term *oncornavirus*.

Linear energy transfer (LET)   The amount of radiation energy delivered to tissue per unit of path length by a charged particle. The magnitude of LET is thus a measure of tissue damage caused by radiotherapy.

Lipids   Cellular components that are insoluble in water but soluble in organic solvents (such as chloroform, ether, and benzene). They include fats (esters of fatty acids with glycerol), waxes (esters of fatty acids with monohydroxy aliphatic alcohols), fatty oils, cholesterol, and related compounds. Lipids are the major component of cellular membranes.

Lipoma   A benign *tumor* arising in fatty tissue.

Liposarcoma   A malignant *tumor* arising in fatty tissue.

Lucké's virus   A *herpesvirus* that causes *adenocarcinomas* in frog kidneys.

Lymph   A pale, coagulable fluid that resembles the plasma of blood and that contains *leukocytes*.

Lymphangioma   A benign *tumor* arising in *lymph* vessels.

Lymph nodes   Masses of lymphatic tissue, 1 to 25 millimeters long and often bean-shaped, that are intercalated in the course of *lymph* vessels. They are more or less well organized by a connective tissue capsule and membranes into nodules and medullary cords, which produce *lymphocytes*, and into lymph filters, which permit *phagocytosis* by *reticuloendothelial* cells and *macrophages*.

Lymphoblast   An immediate *lymphocyte*.

Lymphoblastic leukemia   Lymphocytic *leukemia.*

Lymphocyte   See *leukocytes, T lymphocyte,* and *B lymphocyte.*

Lymphocytic leukemia   See *leukemia.*

Lymphoma   A malignant disease in which abnormal numbers of *lymphocytes* are produced by the spleen and *lymph nodes.* These immature lymphocytes generally aggregate in the lymphoid tissues. *Hodgkin's disease* is the best-known form of lymphoma. Lymphomas account for about 5.4 percent of human malignancies.

Lymphosarcoma   A general term for *lymphomas* other than *Hodgkin's disease.*

Macrophages   Large, mobile cells derived from *monocytes.* Their primary function, like that of *neutrophils,* is *phagocytosis,* which may be followed by degradation of the ingested material. They also ingest neutrophils following tissue damage or infections. Macrophages probably play an accessory role in the processing of *antigens.*

Malignant transformation   See *transformation.*

Mammography   Low-voltage *x-ray* examination of the breasts to detect *tumors.* The image is recorded on conventional x-ray film.

Marek's disease   An infectious *lymphoma* of chickens caused by a *herpesvirus* known as Marek's disease virus. Some evidence suggests that a *type C RNA virus* may also be involved. The disease can be prevented by vaccination with a turkey herpesvirus that is immunologically similar to Marek's disease virus but not pathogenic in either species.

Mast cell   *Basophil.*

Mastectomy   A surgical procedure for removal of breast *tumors.* In a segmental mastectomy, also known as a "lumpectomy," the tumor and a varying—but small—amount of surrounding tissue is removed. In a simple mastectomy, also known as a total mastectomy, the entire breast is removed. In a modified radical mastectomy, the entire breast, the *lymph nodes* in the area, and the associated fatty tissues are removed. In a radical mastectomy, also known as a Halsted radical mastectomy, the entire breast, the lymph nodes, the fatty tissues, and the underlying chest muscles are removed. There is little agreement among physicians about which is the best procedure.

Maytansine   An experimental antitumor agent isolated from *Maytenus buchananii.*

Melanoma   A malignant tumor of pigment-forming cells in the skin or the retina of the eyes.

6-Mercaptopurine   An *antimetabolite* that is a structural analog of hypoxanthine. 6-Mercaptopurine is converted by intracellular enzymes to a *nucleotide*, thioinosine monophosphate, that interferes with the production of adenosine monophosphate and guanosine monophosphate. It thus inhibits the synthesis of DNA.

Mesothelioma   A malignant *tumor* arising in the mesothelial cells that line joints and the body cavities.

Metastasis   The process in which malignant cells detach themselves from a *tumor* and establish a new tumor (called secondary cancer) at a remote site within the host. This process reflects both the lessened cohesiveness of cells within a tumor and the capacity of malignant cells to sustain themselves while floating freely in the blood stream or *lymph* vessels.

Methotrexate   Also known as amethopterin. An *antimetabolite* that is a structural analog of *folic acid.* It inhibits the enzyme folic acid reductase, and thus interferes with the synthesis of DNA and RNA.

Methyl-CCNU   A *nitrosourea* used as an *alkylating agent* in the treatment of *tumors.*

Microsomal mixed-function oxidases   A family of enzymes, found primarily in *microsomes,* that oxidize a wide variety of molecules foreign to the cell for detoxification. Oxidation makes the molecules more polar, and thus more soluble, and provides a point of attachment for sugars and other molecules that help solubilize the foreign chemical so that it can be excreted.

Microsomes   A group of structures, composed primarily of intracellular membranes, that can be isolated by centrifugation, and that comprise about 15 to 20 percent of the total mass of the cell. They have a high content of lipids and of various enzymes. They are active, among other things, in the biosynthesis of phosphatides, glucuronides, and ascorbic acid; in metabolism of 6-carbon sugars; in *steroid* biosynthesis; at certain points in the synthesis of glycerides, phospholipids, and *glycolipids*; and in the detoxification of foreign chemicals

Microtubules   Energy-transducing systems within the cell that are generally used where a pushing force is needed, as in the motion of sperm tails and cilia and in spindle formation and nuclear division during *mitosis.*

Microwave hypothermia   The application of microwave energy in the therapy of *tumors.* Limited experimental evidence suggests not only that microwave energy can kill tumors, but also that it can potentiate the action of conventional radiation.

Migration inhibition factor (MIF) An unidentified substance released by *T lymphocytes* after they react with *antigens* to which they have been sensitized. MIF immobilizes *macrophages* at the site of an injury, infection, or tumor. Immobilized macrophages may destroy foreign or injured cells.

Mithramycin An antitumor *antibiotic*. It is thought to act by binding to cellular DNA, thereby inhibiting the synthesis of RNA.

Mitomycin C An antitumor *antibiotic* isolated from *Streptomyces caespitosus* (griseovinacesus). It is thought to act by binding to DNA to inhibit its replication.

Mitosis The process by which most cells divide to produce two new cells. The main events of mitosis are: duplication of the *chromosomes*; disappearance of the nucleus and nucleolus; formation of the mitotic spindle; separation and migration of the chromosome sets to opposite ends of the cell; restoration of the original condition of the nucleus; and cleavage of the cell into two complete cells.

Molecular hybridization A technique for determining if identical or similar sequences of nucleic acids (homologies) exist between two specimens of DNA or one specimen of DNA and one of RNA.

Monocyte   A type of *leukocyte* in which the nucleus is large and kidney-shaped and the *cytoplasm* contains fine granules. Monocytes are formed in the *bone marrow* and by organs of the *reticuloendothelial system*. They are generally considered to be immature *macrophages* which migrate from the bloodstream and mature into macrophages at the site of injury or infection.

Morphology   The various features of the form and structure of an organism or any of its parts.

Mouse leukemia viruses   A family of *type C RNA viruses* that cause *leukemias* and certain *sarcomas* in mice; they include the Gross, Moloney, Friend, and Rauscher strains. They have generally been isolated from inbred mice having a high incidence of spontaneous lymphoid leukemia.

Mouse mammary tumor virus (*MMTV*)   Also known as the Bittner virus. A *type B RNA virus* that causes breast *tumors* in mice with a certain genetic and hormonal constitution.

Multiple myeloma   A malignant *tumor* thought to arise in *bone marrow*. It is characterized by greatly increased numbers of abnormal plasma cells and the destruction of healthy bone tissue, and is usually associated with anemia, an abnormal immunoglobulin in the blood, and *Bence-Jones protein* in the urine.

Mutagen   Any agent that induces a mutation—a relatively permanent change in the *genome* that is apparent either as a physical change in *chromosome* structure or as a fundamental change in *gene* products or expression. A mutation can occur in either germ cells or *somatic* cells, but only a change in a germ cell will be transmitted to future generations by sexual reproduction.

Myeloblast   A large, mononuclear, nongranular cell of the *bone marrow* that is a precursor of myelocytes, which in turn are precursors of *granulocytes*.

Myelocytic leukemia   See *leukemia*.

Myelogenous leukemia   Myelocytic *leukemia*.

Myeloma   A malignant *tumor* arising in cells of the *bone marrow*.

Myxoma   A benign *tumor* arising in embryonic connective tissue.

Myxosarcoma   A malignant *tumor* arising in embryonic connective tissue.

Myxoviruses   A family of RNA *viruses* that includes influenza viruses, hemagglutinating viruses, and the subgroup of *paramyxoviruses*. The RNA *genome* of myxoviruses has a mass of about 2 to 8×10^6 daltons and is encapsulated in a lipoprotein envelope. Myxoviruses have not been shown to cause *tumors* in any species.

Nasopharyngeal carcinoma   A malignant *tumor* arising in the nasal cavity, pharynx, and oral cavity.

Neoplasia   Cancer.

Neoplasm   A malignant *tumor*.

Neoplastic   Of or relating to malignant *tumors*.

Neuraminidase   An enzyme that splits the linkage between *sialic acid* and mucin, a polysaccharide. Since the membrane *antigens* of many *tumor* cells appear to be masked by a heavy coat of sialic acid, some scientists think that treatment with neuraminidase unmasks the antigens.

Neuroblastoma   A malignant *tumor* arising from primitive nerve cells in the *adrenal gland*. It is the most common tumor of infants.

Neutrophil   Also known as polymorphonuclear neutrophilic *leukocyte*. The major type of *granulocyte* in the blood. A mature neutrophil has a half-life of about 6.6 hours in the blood stream. It contains many pink-staining granules that are the major source of enzymes used for the killing of bacteria following *phagocytosis*. Neutrophils are primarily involved in continuous defense against inflammatory infections caused by bacteria and other parasites.

Nitrogen mustard   Also known as mechlorethamine or Mustargen. A chemical, originally manufactured as a gas warfare agent, used as an *alkylating agent* in the treatment of *tumors*.

$$CH_3-N \begin{cases} CH_2CH_2Cl \\ CH_2CH_2Cl \end{cases}$$

Nitrosamines   A group of chemicals formed by the action of nitrous acid on primary or secondary (mono- or disubstituted) amines and containing the functional group =N—N=O. Many alkyl nitrosamines are powerful *carcinogens.*

Nitrosoureas   A family of *alkylating agents,* including *BCNU, CCNU,* and *methyl-CCNU,* used in the treatment of tumors. They represent one of the few classes of antitumor agents able to cross the blood-brain barrier and attack malignant cells in the central nervous system. They are also powerful *carcinogens.*

Nonvirion antigens   Substances—generally proteins or *glycoproteins*—that are produced by a *virus* during infection of a cell but that are not themselves either structural components of the virus or a normal constituent of the cell. The host organism will thus consider them to be foreign and will produce *antibodies* against them.

Nucleoid   The nucleic acid core and associated proteins of a *virus.*

Nucleophilic   Electron-rich; capable of attacking electron-deficient (*electrophilic*) centers in other molecules. Typical nucleophiles include amines, halide ions, hydroxide ion, and carboxylate anions.

Nucleoside   The combination of a purine (adenine, guanine, hypoxanthine) or pyrimidine (uracil, cytosine, thymine) base and a sugar, either D-deoxyribose in the case of DNA or D-ribose in the case of RNA.

Nucleotide   A *nucleoside* in which the sugar is esterified with a phosphate group.

Occult carcinoma   A small *carcinoma* that is asymptomatic or an asymptomatic primary *tumor* that gives rise to metastases.

Oncogene   A *gene* that contains information sufficient for the initiation of a *tumor.* The once-popular theory that all mammalian and avian cells contain such a gene has been largely discredited.

Oncogenesis   The initiation of *tumor* formation.

Oncogenic   *Tumor* causing.

Oncology   The study of the causes, development, characteristics, and treatment of *tumors.*

Oncornavirus   An *oncogenic* RNA virus. The term is generally used to describe the *type A, type B,* and *type C RNA viruses,* even though not all of them have been shown to be oncogenic.

Osteogenic sarcoma   A malignant *tumor* composed of bone cells.

Osteoma   A benign *tumor* composed of bone cells.

Papilloma   A benign *tumor* arising from skin or mucous membranes (the coverings of passages or cavities that lead to the interior of the body).

Papovaviruses   A family of DNA viruses that includes papilloma viruses, polyoma viruses, vacuolating viruses, and human wart viruses. The DNA of papovaviruses has a mass of about 2 to 4×10^6 daltons. Some papovaviruses, such as the *SV 40* and polyoma viruses, produce tumors in laboratory animals. Certain papillomas—large, localized, fleshy tumors with a horny surface on the neck and shoulders of rabbits—produced by members of this family occur in vivo.

Pap smear   A section of cells which have flaked off the interior of the uterine cervix that is microscopically examined to determine if a *tumor* is present. The Pap smear is a very effective means for discovering cervical tumors that cannot be discerned by other methods; its use has lowered the death rate from cervical cancer by 38 percent in the last 15 years, even though only about half of all women in the United States are tested at regular intervals.

Paramyxoviruses   A family of RNA *viruses* that includes mumps virus, measles virus, parainfluenza viruses (which cause respiratory infections, not influenza), and Newcastle disease virus. The RNA core of paramyxoviruses has a mass of about 8×10^6 daltons and is enclosed in a lipoprotein envelope. Paramyxoviruses have not been shown to cause *tumors* in any species.

Parenchyma   The functional cells of an organ or the abnormal (malignant) cells that compose a *tumor*—as opposed to the supporting tissues, or *stroma*.

Phagocytosis   The process by which certain cells (phagocytes)—especially *monocytes* and *neutrophils*—engulf and sometimes destroy tissue debris and invading bacteria. It can be viewed as a sequence of three events: (1) Chemotaxis, the attraction of the phagocytes to the site of injury or infection. Chemotaxis is related to the combination of *antigens* with specific, sensitized *T lymphocytes*. (2) Engulfment of the bacteria or other cell by formation of a vacuole within the *cytoplasm* of the phagocyte. (3) The actual killing of the bacteria, accomplished when certain phagocyte granules (lysosomes) fuse with the vacuole and release lysing enzymes into it. The cell fragments thus formed are subsequently eliminated from the cell and, in many cases, passed on to the appropriate *lymphocytes* for *cell-mediated* or *humoral immune* responses.

Phenylalanine mustard   Two *alkylating agents* used in the treatment of *tumors* and distinguished by the asymmetry of the amino acid moiety. L-Phenylalanine mustard is also known as Melphalan or L-sarcolysine. D-Phenylalanine mustard is also known as Medphalan or D-sarcolysine.

$$HOOC\underset{H_2N}{\overset{}{\diagdown}}CHCH_2-\overset{}{\bigcirc}-N\overset{CH_2CH_2Cl}{\underset{CH_2CH_2Cl}{<}}$$

Philadelphia chromosome   A *chromosome*, number 22, in *lymphocytes* from patients with chronic myelocytic *leukemia* which is shorter than its counterpart in cells from healthy tissues. The Philadelphia chromosome is found in more than 90 percent of such patients.

Pion   A pi minus meson, a negatively charged particle with a mass about 273 times that of an electron. Pions have a mean lifetime of about 2.54×10^{-8} seconds, decaying first to muons, then to electrons. They have shown some promise for use in the radiotherapy of *tumors.*

Pituitary gland   Also known as the hypophysis. A small organ, located below the brain, that is responsible for the synthesis and release of at least nine different *hormones.*

Plasmapheresis   A technique, generally involving centrifugation, for removing desired components from blood and returning the rest to the donor.

Platelets   Also known as thrombocytes. Fragments of megakaryocyte cytoplasm produced in the *bone marrow* and involved in the initiation of blood coagulation and contraction of the clot. Their concentration in the blood is generally about 250,000 per cubic millimeter.

Polycyclic aromatic hydrocarbons   Complex hydrocarbons which are made up of several fused benzene rings.

Prednisone   A synthetic *steroid hormone* used as an antitumor agent.

Preinvasive carcinoma   *Carcinoma-in-situ.*

Procarbazine   An antitumor agent whose mechanism of action is not clear. It is also carcinogenic.

Prolactin   A *hormone*, secreted by the *pituitary gland,* that is required for lactation. It has also been implicated in the development of mammary *tumors* in mice.

Protovirus theory   A theory that mammalian and avian cells contain a particular type of *virogene*, the protovirus, that directs the production of an RNA copy of certain segments of the cellular *genome*, and then packages the copy and an *RNA-directed DNA polymerase* in a particle that is able to infect the nucleus of a neighboring cell or reinfect the nucleus of the cell of origin. The protovirus, in effect, provides a method for inter- and intracellular transfer of information from DNA to RNA to DNA. It has been suggested as a source for the generation of oncogenic information within a cell.

Provirus   A DNA copy of the *genome* of an RNA *tumor virus.* This copy serves as a template for the production of more virus particles and is thus an intermediate in viral replication. It is also a form of the RNA genome that can be *integrated* into the host cell's genome.

Proximate carcinogen   See *ultimate carcinogen.*

Pseudotumor   A nonmalignant mass of tissue, such as a callus or a *cyst.*

Rad   The unit used to express the absorbed dose of any ionizing radiation; the amount of energy imparted to matter by ionizing particles per unit mass of irradiated material.

Radical mastectomy   See *mastectomy.*

Radioimmunoassay (RIA)   Also known as competitive binding assay or saturation analysis. A very sensitive technique for measuring small concentrations of a substance in biological fluids. In the assay, radioactive-labeled *antigens* compete with antigens in the fluid for binding sites on specially prepared *antibodies.*

RD-114   An *endogenous xenotropic virus* of cats. It was once thought to be a human cancer virus.

Recognition factor   A protein (alphaglobulin) that combines with certain types of foreign matter to mark it for destruction by *macrophages.*

Remission   A period of good health occurring after the onset of cancer and associated with a reduction in the size of the *tumor.* Remission may occur spontaneously or be induced by therapy, but it should not be confused with cure as it more often represents only a temporary quiescence of the malignancy.

Reticuloendothelial system   A network of *monocytes* and *macrophages* distributed throughout the body in the blood, spleen, liver, *lymph nodes,* connective tissues, and *bone marrow.* The cells of this system are involved in the *phagocytosis* of tissue debris and bacteria, storage of fatty materials, scavenging of worn-out red blood cells, and the metabolism of iron and pigments.

Reticuloendothelioma   A malignant *tumor* arising in cells of the *reticuloendothelial system.*

Reticuloendotheliosis   *Hyperplasia* of cells of the *reticuloendothelial system.*

Reverse transcriptase   *RNA-directed DNA polymerase.*

Rhabdomyoma   A benign *tumor* arising in striated muscle.

Rhabdomyosarcoma   A combined *sarcoma* and *rhabdomyoma.*

Rhabdosarcoma   A *sarcoma* containing striated muscle fibers.

Ribonuclease   An enzyme that attacks and depolymerizes RNA.

Rifampicin   A derivative of *rifamycin SV* that is used to treat tuber-culosis and that may be a potential antitumor agent.

Rifamycin SV   An *antibiotic* isolated from *Streptomyces mediterranei.* It is the progenitor of a family of compounds that have shown potential both as antiviral agents and as antitumor agents. They are thought to act by inhibiting DNA polymerases.

RNA-directed DNA polymerase   Also known as reverse transcrip-tase. An enzyme that mediates the synthesis of DNA, using an RNA template. It is found primarily in *oncornaviruses* or in cells infected by them.

RNA tumor virus   *Oncornavirus.*

Rous sarcoma virus   A *type C RNA virus.* The Rous sarcoma virus was one of the first viruses shown to cause tumors in animals. Its primary host is chickens, but it has also been shown to cause tumors in hamsters, rabbits, and monkeys. Subsequent work has shown that at least some strains of it are defective; these can replicate or produce a tumor only in the presence of a "helper" virus, the Rous-associated virus, that supplies the outer coat of the viral particle.

Rubidazone   An antitumor *antibotic* that is a synthetically prepared analog of *daunorubicin*. It is believed to act by binding to cellular DNA to block the production of RNA.

Sarcolysine   *Phenylalanine mustard.*

Sarcoma   A malignant *tumor* arising from derivatives of embryonal mesoderm. These include: the lining of the body cavity; the circulatory system; certain parts of the excretory system; muscle; bone; teeth (except the enamel); mesenchymal tissues, such as cartilage, connective tissue, adipose tissue, and tendon; blood; and the reproductive organs. *Leukemias* and *lymphomas* can thus be considered subgroups of sarcomas. Sarcomas (not including leukemias and lymphomas) account for about 2 percent of human malignancies.

Segmental mastectomy   See *mastectomy.*

Seminoma   A malignant *tumor* of the testis; it is derived from germinal *epithelium* that has not differentiated to cells of either male or female type.

Sialic acids   N-Acyl derivatives of neuraminic acid, a 9-carbon amino sugar. The most common is N-acetylneuraminic acid.

Simian sarcoma virus   A *type C RNA virus* that produces a *leukemia-*like disease in monkeys.

Somatic cell   Any cell other than a germ (egg or sperm) cell.

Squamous-cell carcinoma   Also called *epithelioma,* a malignant *tumor* composed of flat cells arising from the *epithelium.*

Steroids   A family of compounds sharing the cyclopentanoperhy-drophenanthrene skeleton. This group includes cholesterol, ergos-terol, the bile acids, the sex *hormones,* the D-vitamins, and the cardiac glycosides. Some steroids are useful as antitumor agents.

Streptozotocin   An antitumor *antibiotic* isolated from *Streptomyces achromogenes* that is a potential *alkylating agent.* It is one of the few antitumor agents that do not suppress synthesis of *leukocytes* in the *bone marrow.*

Stroma   The supporting network of connective tissue and blood vessels in a normal organ or a *tumor.* (Compare *parenchyma.*)

SV40   Also known as simian vacuolating virus. A DNA *virus* of the *papovavirus* family that produces seemingly inapparent infections in monkeys, especially rhesus monkeys, and that is a common contaminant of monkey cell cultures. It has been shown to produce *tumors* in hamsters and to *transform* cultured monkey cells. Tumors caused by SV40 exhibit a specific *antigen* associated with the virus and known as T-antigen.

Syncytium-forming virus   An RNA *virus* that causes cells to fuse into large masses. Syncytium-forming viruses contain an *RNA-directed*

DNA polymerase and replicate through a DNA intermediate, but they have never been shown to cause *tumors.*

Teratocarcinoma A malignant *tumor* arising from germ cells in the ovary or testis.

Teratoma A benign *tumor* arising in the ovary or testis.

Thalicarpine A potential antitumor agent isolated from *Thalictrum dasycarpum.* Its mechanism of action is unknown.

Thermography The use of an infrared detector to produce a photograph of the heat pattern of a tissue, particularly breasts, for detection of *tumors.* Tumors appear as hot spots in the thermogram because of their altered metabolism or increased blood supply. Thermography alleviates the hazards associated with x-irradiation, but it is not specific for cancer.

6-Thioguanine An *antimetabolite* that is a structural analog of guanine. It is converted by intracellular enzymes to a *nucleotide,* 6-thioguanine monophosphate, that interferes with the synthesis of other nucleotides and thus inhibits the synthesis of DNA and RNA.

Thio-TEPA   Triethylene thiophosphoramide. An *alkylating agent* used in the treatment of *tumors*.

$$
\begin{array}{c}
CH_2 \qquad\quad S \qquad\quad CH_2 \\
| \quad\ \diagdown \quad\ || \quad\ \diagup \quad\ | \\
\qquad\quad N-P-N \\
| \quad\ \diagup \quad\ | \quad\ \diagdown \quad\ | \\
CH_2 \qquad\quad N \qquad\quad CH_2 \\
\diagup\ \diagdown \\
H_2C \longrightarrow CH_2
\end{array}
$$

T lymphocytes   Also known as thymus-dependent lymphocytes. A group of *lymphocytes* that are involved in *cell-mediated immunity*, rejection of grafts, delayed *hypersensitivity* reactions, and graft-versus-host reactions. T lymphocyte precursors from the *bone marrow* and other lymphoid tissues accumulate in the thymus, where they become thymocytes. The thymocytes proliferate from the cortex of the thymus and move inward to the medullary region, where they mature. They then enter the circulating pool of lymphocytes and are called T lymphocytes; they account for 70 to 80 percent of circulating lymphocytes. There are at least two distinct populations of T lymphocytes: One is produced slowly and has a half-life of 100 to 200 days; the other is produced rapidly and has a half-life of 3 to 4 days. The difference between the two is not fully understood.

Total mastectomy   See *mastectomy.*

Transfer factor   A conjugate of nucleic acid and polypeptide, isolated from *B lymphocytes,* that apparently transfers *cell-mediated immunity* from one individual to another. Transfer factor from individuals who have recovered from a specific type of *tumor,* for example, could theoretically be used to treat others with the same tumor. It is thought to act by somehow activating the recipient's *lymphocytes.*

Transformation   The conversion of a healthy cell to a malignant one, either in culture or in an organism. Transformation may be initiated by chemicals, radiation, or *viruses,* or may occur spontaneously. With cultured cells, transformation is associated with the appearance of a set of specific changes that are thought to represent malignancy.

Triethylenemelamine   An *alkylating agent* used in the treatment of tumors.

Tripdiolide   A potential antitumor agent isolated from *Tripterygium wilfordii.* Its mechanism of action is unknown.

Trypsin   A highly active proteolytic enzyme found in many body tissues. It cleaves the amide carbon–nitrogen bond between certain amino acids in a protein.

Tumor   An anomalous tissue mass in the body, derived from preexisting cells, that serves no purpose and grows independently of surrounding tissue. Most tumors must contain more than 1 billion (10^9) cells before they can be discerned clinically. Benign tumors remain localized, are usually slow growing, and produce symptoms only when they become large enough to interfere mechanically with surrounding structures. The cells of benign tumors resemble adult body cells, and the tumor generally does not recur when it is completely removed. Malignant (cancerous) tumors invade surrounding tissues, disseminate to other parts of the body (*metastasis*), produce such symptoms as *cachexia,* and are generally fatal. The cells of malignant tumors resemble embryonic cells. The *parenchyma* of a tumor is the abnormal cells, while the *stroma* is the supporting network of connective tissues and blood vessels. The cause of most tumors is unknown.

Tumor angiogenesis factor (TAF)   A substance secreted by *tumors* to stimulate the formation of blood vessels and thus enhance their own blood supply.

Tumor-associated antigens   Membrane components that are found only in malignant cells. Many scientists think that most *tumors* contain such *antigens,* but isolating and identifying them has proved to be a major problem. Identification of tumor-associated antigens that are specific for particular types of tumors would provide a good method for the early detection of cancer.

Type A RNA viruses   A small group of viruslike particles that have not been shown to be infectious, have not been found outside the confines of cells, and have not been shown to be oncogenic. They are encapsulated by a protein shell rather than by a lipid-containing membrane. Type A particles found in cellular *cytoplasm* are believed to be immature forms of *type B RNA viruses,* to which they are immunologically similar; those found in cisternae (reservoirs for lymph and other body fluids) are suspected to be immature *type C RNA viruses.*

Type B RNA viruses   A family of RNA *viruses* whose principal member is the *mouse mammary tumor virus.* They are very similar to *type C RNA viruses,* differing primarily in the size of internal proteins (and thus the size of the core) and in the size and spacing of *glycoprotein* spikes on the surface of the viral envelope.

Type C RNA viruses   The largest family of animal *tumor viruses.* Most type C RNA viruses are oncogenic, causing mainly *leukemias, lymphomas,* and *sarcomas* in a variety of species. They are larger than most other RNA viruses; their *genome* has a mass of about 12×10^6 daltons. They also contain more species of proteins—most important, an *RNA-directed DNA polymerase*—and nucleic acids. Types A, B, and C RNA viruses are thought to replicate in the nucleus of a cell, unlike most other RNA viruses, which replicate in the cytoplasm.

Ultimate carcinogen   A metabolic derivative of a chemical *carcinogen* that actually reacts with some component of the cell to initiate *transformation.* The derivative formed immediately prior to the ultimate carcinogen is known as the proximate carcinogen. The carcinogen 2-acetylaminofluorene, for example, is first oxidized to N-hydroxy-2-acetylaminofluorene, which is a proximate carcinogen. This compound may then be converted into a sulfuric acid ester which is one of the ultimate carcinogens that reacts with cellular components.

Vertical transmission The transfer of a *virus* from parent to progeny during reproduction. This can occur by *integration* of the virus into parental germ cells; alternatively, the virus could simply be very closely associated with the DNA of parental germ cells.

Vinblastine An antitumor alkaloid isolated from periwinkle (*Vinca rosea* Linn.). It is believed to be an inhibitor of *mitosis*, destroying the mitotic spindle and thus halting cell division.

R = CH₃

Vincristine An antitumor alkaloid isolated from periwinkle (*Vinca rosea* Linn.). It is believed to be an inhibitor of *mitosis*, destroying the mitotic spindle and thus halting cell division. Its structure is the same as that of *vinblastine* with R=CHO. Vincristine sulfate is also known as Oncovin.

Virion The complete *virus* particle.

Virogene A *gene* that is the template for the production of a *virus*. Many scientists now think that all mammalian and avian cells contain a virogene, but its purpose is still a subject of debate.

Virus One of a group of minute infectious agents requiring living cells for their replication and containing either DNA or RNA but not both. The mature infectious unit (*virion*) usually contains proteins, and sometimes contains *glycoproteins*, lipids, and polyamines. Some viruses are encapsulated in a lipid-containing membrane or envelope. Viruses differ from other microorganisms in that they lack genetic information for generation of energy and they do not divide by binary fission.

Warburg effect The unexplained observation that many *tumor* cells rely on *glycolysis* for energy production to a much greater extent than do normal cells.

Wilms' tumor Also called embryonal carcinosarcoma. A malignant *tumor* arising in the kidney of children. It contains elements of both *carcinomas* and *sarcomas*.

Xenotropic viruses *Endogenous viruses* that do not, under most conditions, replicate in the species of origin. The distinction between xenotropic viruses and ecotropic viruses (those that do replicate in the species of origin) is a very fine one, and it is possible that endogenous ecotropic viruses are simply endogenous xenotropic viruses that have mutated slightly after their exposure to the chemical agents used to activate *latent viruses*. Xenotropic viruses have so far been isolated from cats, chickens, hamsters, mice, rats, and pigs, but are believed to be present in all mammalian and avian species.

Xeroradiography A technique for low-voltage *x-ray* examination of the breast to detect *tumors*. Xeroradiography involves less exposure to x-rays than does conventional *mammography* because the image is recorded on a very sensitive metal plate coated with a semiconductor such as selenium.

X-rays Electromagnetic radiation with wavelengths in the range 10^{-11} to 10^{-8} meters.

Selected Readings

ETIOLOGY

1. ELIZABETH C. MILLER AND JAMES A. MILLER, Approaches to the mechanisms and control of chemical carcinogenesis, in: *Environment and Cancer*, Williams and Wilkins Company, Baltimore (1972).
2. PAUL O. P. TS'O AND JOSEPH A. DIPAOLO, eds., *Chemical Carcinogenesis*, Marcel Dekker, New York (1974). Two volumes.
3. KEEN A. RAFFERTY, Herpesviruses and cancer, *Scientific American* **229**, 26 (October, 1973).
4. FRED RAPP, Herpesviruses and cancer, *Advances in Cancer Research* **19**, 265 (1974).
5. HOWARD M. TEMIN, The cellular and molecular biology of RNA tumour viruses, especially avian leukosis-sarcoma viruses and their relatives, *Advances in Cancer Research* **19** (1974).
6. GEORGE J. TODARO AND ROBERT J. HUEBNER, The viral oncogene hypothesis: New evidence, *Proceedings of the National Academy of Sciences U.S.A.* **69**, 1009 (1972).
7. KARL ERIK HELLSTRÖM AND INGEGERD HELLSTRÖM, The role of cell-mediated immunity in control and growth of tumors, in: *Clinical Immunobiology*, Vol. II, R. Good and F. Bach, eds., Academic Press, New York (1974), p. 233.
8. RICHMOND PREHN, Immunological surveillance: Pro and con, in: *Clinical Immunobiology*, Vol. II, R. Good and F. Bach, eds., Academic Press, New York (1974), p. 191.
9. THOMAS A. WALDMANN, WARREN STROBER, AND R. MICHAEL BLAESE, Immunodeficiency disease and malignancy, *Annals of Internal Medicine* **77**, 605 (1972).

BIOCHEMISTRY

1. MAX M. BURGER, Surface properties of neoplastic cells, *Hospital Practice* **8**, 55 (July, 1973).
2. GARTH L. NICOLSON, Factors influencing the dynamic display of lectin binding sites on normal and transformed cell surfaces, in: *Control of Proliferation in Animal Cells*, B. Clarkson and R. Baserga, eds., Cold Spring Harbor Laboratory, New York (1974), p. 81.

3. J. H. COGGIN, JR., AND N. G. ANDERSON, Cancer, differentiation, and embryonic antigens: Some central problems, *Advances in Cancer Research* **19**, 105 (1974).

THERAPY

1. JOSEPH H. BURCHENAL AND STEPHEN K. CARTER, New cancer chemotherapeutic agents, *Cancer* **30**, 1639 (1972).
2. VINCENT T. DEVITA, JR., GEORGE P. CANELLOS, AND JOHN H. MOXLEY III, A decade of combination chemotherapy of advanced Hodgkin's disease, *Cancer* **30**, 1495 (1972).
3. IRWIN H. KRAKOFF, The present status of cancer chemotherapy, *Medical Clinics of North America* **55**, 683 (1971).
4. HERBERT J. RAPP, Immunotherapy of cancer, in: *Current Research in Oncology*, C. B. Anfinsen *et al.*, eds., Academic Press, New York (1973).
5. JOHN E. HEALEY, JR., ed., *Ecology of the Cancer Patient: Proceedings of Thrree Interdisciplinary Conferences on Rehabilitation of the Patient with Cancer,* Interdisciplinary Communication Associates, Inc., Washington, D.C. (1970).
6. *Proceedings of the American Cancer Society's National Conference on Human Values and Cancer,* American Cancer Society, Inc., New York (1973).

SPECIFIC CANCERS

1. BRIAN MACMAHON, PHILIP COLE, AND JAMES BROWN, Etiology of human breast cancer: A review, *Journal of the National Cancer Institute* **50**, 21 (1973).
2. BERNARD FISHER, The surgical dilemma in the primary therapy of invasive breast cancer: A critical appraisal, *Current Problems in Surgery*, p. 3 (October, 1970).
3. JOSEPH V. SIMONE, Acute lymphocytic leukemia in childhood, *Seminars in Hematology* **11**, 25 (1974).

GENERAL

1. JAMES F. HOLLAND AND EMIL FREI III, eds., *Cancer Medicine*, Lea and Febiger, Philadelphia (1973).
2. JAMES D. WATSON, *Molecular Biology of the Gene*, W. A. Benjamin, New York (1972).
3. *Advances in Cancer Research*, Vol. 1 through the current volume, Academic Press, New York.
4. FREDERICK F. BECKER, ed., *Cancer, A Comprehensive Treatise*, Plenum Publishing Corporation, New York (1975).

Index

Abelov, G. I., 92
Ablashi, Dharam, 26, 35
2-Acetylaminofluorene, 13, 14, 17, 236
N-Acetylglucosamine, 210
N-Acetylneuraminic acid, 231
Actinomycin D, 113, 116, 119, 120,
   125, 128, 192, 195
Acute Leukemia Group B, 178
Adamson, Richard H., 92
Adenocarcinoma, 193
Adenoma, 193
Adenoviruses, 24, 193
Adjuvant chemotherapy, see Chemother-
   apy
Adrenal glands, 157, 161, 164
Adriamycin, 114, 116, 121, 125, 127,
   128, 179, 193, 195
Aflatoxin, 194
Agglutination, 77-82, 194, 209
Agriculture, Department of, 34
Ainsworth, Thomas H., 98
Alabama, University of, 144
Alkylating agents, 11, 16, 113, 114, 116,
   117, 124, 128, 194, 198, 200, 201
Alpha-fetoprotein, 89, 91-93, 194
Ambrus, Julian L., 7
American Cancer Society, 4, 88, 99, 145,
   146, 155, 161, 181-185, 188, 191, 240
American Health Foundation, 10
Ames, Bruce N., 12, 21
Amethopterin, see Methotrexate
Aminopterin, 175, 194, 209

Anaplasia, 6, 91, 195
Anderson, David, 156
Anderson Hospital and Tumor Institute,
   M. D., 17, 106, 115, 121, 131, 132,
   144, 152, 153, 156, 175
Anderson, Norman G., 90, 91, 239
Androgens, 113, 128, 164, 195
Angioma, 195
Angiosarcoma, 195
Antibiotics, 117, 119, 125, 127, 128,
   192, 193, 195, 198, 201, 205, 222,
   230-232
Antibodies, 26, 27, 30, 31, 56, 60-63,
   168, 195, 198, 199, 213, 214, 225,229
Antigens, 54, 56, 58, 63, 89, 90, 195,
   198, 202, 213, 214, 219, 222, 224,
   229,
   early, 27, 31, 32
   fetal, 88-94, 118, 208
   nonvirion, 30-32, 225
   nuclear, 31, 32
   shedding, 61, 62
   tumor-associated, 28, 33, 44, 54, 55,
      60-62, 64, 66, 90, 94, 98, 119, 131,
      136, 138, 232, 235
   virus-specific, 28, 35
Antimetabolite, 118, 120, 124, 128,
   129, 175, 194-197, 199, 202, 209,
   220, 233
Arabinosylcytosine, 113, 114, 116, 117,
   122, 124, 128, 176, 177, 179, 196
Ara-C, see Arabinosylcytosine